SUNSHINE ROSE

Released on December 8, 2018
Published by StepSister Press, 600 S. Crescent Avenue,
Park Ridge, Illinois, U.S.A., stepsisterpress.org

ISBN: 978-1-7326989-0-1

The views and opinions expressed in this
volume are solely those of the author.

Thank you to our Patreon sponsors for
making this publication possible.

Cover image and lettering by Elana Tenner
of Planet E.T., planetet.com.
Interior layout by StepSister Press.
This book was typeset using Cooper Hewitt and Minion Pro
typefaces and printed on acid-free paper by Ingram Spark.

SUNSHINE ROSE

What My Mother Taught Me about Aging, Alzheimer's, and the End of Life

CAMILLE GRAFER

STEPSISTER
PRESS

Table of Contents

Publisher's Note

Mrs. Grafer, as I knew her, was my very-first-ever-in-the-world-teacher-outside-of-the-home, the first person who tended to my curious little person with every form of care I can imagine: encouragement for my hunger for books and language, correction for my more eccentric vocal disruptions in the cloakroom, and a deep respect for me, a nerd with two left feet, who received all good marks except for a *zero* when it came to throwing a ball. She taught me that it was possible to learn seriously, with a sense of humor.

Imagine my surprise to learn that Mrs. Grafer was an adult human with other concerns, who cared for others. As is so often the case, we children think that our teachers are only there in the form we know, but in fact, it appears that they do other things after school. This book is about some of those other things.

Because this book came to StepSister Press as a publishing company working in very different genres, I naturally questioned how it could fit into the setting created by our other books, and then decided that this particular book demanded a new setting. This setting is a series of books containing the writings of our teachers, my teachers and the teachers of others, with attention to the things they did in school—when they want to write about those—and attention to the many things it seems they must have done at other times. Entitled "Words from Teachers," this series is a loose, simple gesture to initiate what I hope will become an abundant, and perhaps more structured, encounter with the writings and other creations of teachers, where students help to elicit and curate their teachers' words as books. Some readers may notice a connection to the title *Words of My Perfect Teacher*, a work by the 19th-century Tibetan author Patrul Rinpoche. The connection is light but intentional.

For this appreciation of teachers and their many types of work, I am indebted to my former colleagues and superiors at the Museum of Contemporary Art Chicago, some of whom have since moved on to work at other institutions. These dynamic educators cultivated in me the appreciation of teaching as an art form. They include Marissa Reyes, Dominique Enriquez, Lauren Watkins, Lauren Jackson, Lydia Ross, and most intimately, Rachel L. S. Harper, whose love of teaching and teachers is contagious and persistent, like a song you hear once and never forget.

It is important to thank the many readers and contributors who gave their time to this project, including my sisters, Christina M. Heckman and Marianne J. Heckman. They have entertained my queries at all times, offering helpful perspective. The author, in her acknowledgments, will mention a number of names, and I would like to underline her thanks to the community in Park Ridge, Illinois, and in particular at St. Paul of the Cross Church, for encouraging this project and lending their support through photographs and permissions to use their names in telling this story. Elana Tenner breathed new life into the cover design for this project, easing my mind for perhaps the hundredth time in a working relatioship that spans several years.

I would like to thank the author for entrusting this book to an independent publisher on a slow schedule, and for offering these most private lessons in a public forum to help others in what is often a delicate, secret world of family care. This book inspires me personally because it highlights some of the social justice projects active in Catholic communities, and because it takes up what I consider to be a most radical cause: genuine care for others during the later years of their lives. In this way, it unites a world of my youth, a world I little understood, with social concerns I pursued later in life. I think this book will be of tremendous benefit, both as a record of a teacher's life and as a set of recommendations for care. The reader gets to learn seriously, with a sense of humor.

Lastly, this book would not have come into being without the loving editorial stewardship of my mother, Jacqueline U. Heckman, and the quiet support of my father, Philip E. Heckman. They bring 75 years of wisdom to these efforts, and were my very-first-ever-in-the-world-teachers-inside-of-the-home.

Annie Heckman
Toronto, August 23, 2018

Mama Rose at Camille and Richard's home

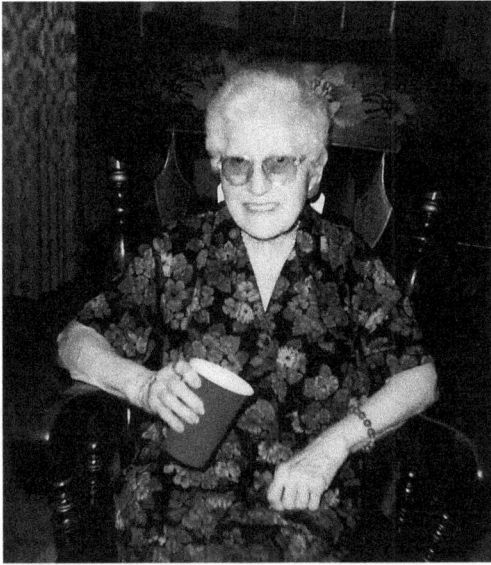

Introduction

In thinking about my reasons for writing this reflection, I found my purpose to be twofold. First, I hoped to be able to help families facing Alzheimer's to understand the disease and its effects, to ease their fears, and to encourage them to understand that the person with this illness needs visitors and, above all, to be loved. Secondly, I wanted to pay tribute to my Mama Rose, who touched so many lives throughout her life and in her battle with Alzheimer's disease.

It is so easy to say, "This person doesn't know if I'm there or not." It becomes easy to turn away from this person who is no longer the loved one you knew, who is now incapable of recognizing what is happening. Perhaps you will need to love more, for you will not get the love back as you did in the past. In some instances, the person with Alzheimer's even gets very violent with those who used to be closest in the past.

You will find many people who don't understand the disease or what's happening. If your parent with Alzheimer's becomes a part of your household, you will need lots of communication within the entire family. If the situation becomes destructive, you need to consider another plan for care. There are many difficult decisions to be made at each stage of the disease.

Along with taking care of your loved one, you must learn how to get information about the money and services that are available. You will need resources, knowledge, and lots of patience with all the paperwork that must be completed and the many phone calls that must be made for services. Often the financial burden falls on the same individual who has assumed responsibility for physical care.

It is important to stay close to your loved one and maintain a sense of humor, even when it is difficult, for their sake as well as your own. You must fight the feelings of sadness, for they will take you away from the person your loved one is now becoming. You must fight the feelings of pity, for they will deny the person dignity. You must fight the feelings of guilt if you can't always cope, for that will be reflected to your loved one as rejection. Fight indifference, for it leaves you empty. If you pass up the opportunity to care, this can leave you without spiritual peace.

So many wonderful souls are sitting alone in nursing homes, hoping to see a visitor. They just want someone to look at them or possibly talk with them. Often they want someone to just smile at them, or someone to share a laugh with them. They are confused and perhaps difficult to be with, but they are very special people. From my experience, I know that I received so much more from these folks than I ever gave them, every day.

You need a great deal of faith in a Creator who loves us. You need to see your caregiver role as one of service and love. The rewards are overwhelming when you seek graces from God, and you will find the strength to get through each day and not view your caregiving as a burden, but as a grace to be cherished. You will find a new relationship with God that will become much more alive and active.

Through all of Mama's illness, I never heard her feel sorry for herself or blame God. She always had a love of God, but during her illness it really became apparent. She always had a prayer on her lips and a smile on her face. I was fortunate that my dear Mama Rose could be an inspiration always and truly be my sunshine.

Mama Rose's graduation photo

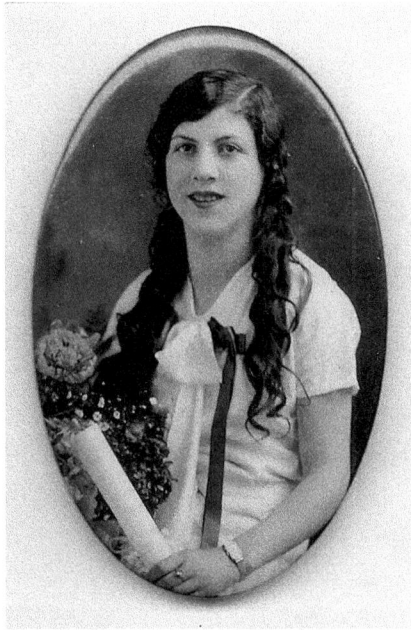

1

Mama Rose

My Mama Rose was born in Chicago on June 5, 1914 to two Italian immigrants, Francisco and Maria, whose marriage had been arranged by their families in Naples. They were beginning an adventure: a new life in America. Grandpa Francisco came first, searching for work and a home in Chicago. When Grandma Maria joined him, she already had their baby boy. They set down their roots in a house on Sangamon and Taylor Streets in Chicago's Little Italy and started a large family of their own. Mama's parents worked hard during those years to survive. They also made sure that they maintained their traditions from the old country. Francisco worked as a pipe maker at Crane Company. Maria's work was in the home, taking care of the household and the children, keeping the family together through prayerful guidance. Mama Rose was the third oldest of seven children, and for a long time, the only girl. The family's world centered on their parish church, Holy Family, and on their neighborhood of Italian friends who, like themselves, came to America to start a new life. Friendships were made with neighbors and they all shared much of their lives, telling story after story of how life had been in Italy and how proud they were to have come to Chicago.

All the neighbors shopped at the grocery store down the street and at the bakery around the corner. The smell of fresh bread wafted down the entire block (I can still to this day remember the wonderful aromas in the neighborhood from the bakery and the neighborhood kitchens). Most of the children on the block went to the school across the street from their homes, Goodrich Public School. During recess, the boys played baseball in the schoolyard and the girls played other games. On free days, the children still played in the neighborhood but helped their families with chores as well. Mama and her siblings went to the parish school, Holy Family, because the parish was the heart of the neighborhood and of their family life. On special days such as a feast of our Blessed Mother, there were religious processions for the Madonna right on Sangamon Street in front of the homes. There would be a huge celebration afterwards with music and the most delicious foods prepared by the parish women and shared by all.

In those days a daughter carried a lot of responsibility for the family. Mama Rose's role was very important because her mother's health started to fail after she lost two children in childbirth. So the responsibility to take over the motherly jobs in the home went to Mama Rose. In those difficult times education was important, but Mama never finished school. It was not an option. While the boys had to have an education, Mama Rose was able to complete school only to the eighth grade like many other girls from immigrant families at that time. She had to educate herself through books. When Mama was in her teens, another boy was born and then the last baby, a girl, her only sister. Mama had more responsibility, but she loved mothering the two little ones.

Mama's routine was not difficult, but it was lonely for a teenager. She had a limited outside life. But she never complained. She enjoyed caring for her family even though it meant that she was not able to go out often. And she also did not want to cause concern by talking about herself. While there was a deep love in the home, feelings were not expressed easily. If there was a problem, no one talked about it. Mama always said she didn't want to be a burden.

Then there was the time of the Depression, a time of poverty. Grandpa Francisco made wine in the basement to be enjoyed at meals. Mama Rose learned quickly how to bake bread and cakes and to cook for a large family of hungry boys as her mother had done with so much talent (Mama always maintained her love of cooking mouth-watering meals throughout her years until she was stricken with Alzheimer's). Mama always loved to work crossword puzzles and to read books. Many times there was only the newspaper to read. Folks sat outside their homes on a warm night sharing stories and laughing. This was Mama's outside life: very simple, compact, lonely, and adventure-free, but happy. She had no social life, but she was always well liked by the people around her, because she was very pleasant even though she was shy.

Mama was 20 years old when a friend introduced her to Anthony Pietrafesa, the man she would eventually marry. He was easy-going and equally shy and quiet. He was a hard worker and a good provider as a laundry man, a good man. He picked up and delivered laundry often to third and fourth floor apartments—later we learned what a strain this had been on his health. He always had a Coke in hand. He was very thin, and yet he worked very hard and seldom complained. Actually, he said very little. Mama used to say, "He needed a little wine to talk and joke." He loved his car, and in his spare time he liked to fool around building wooden objects.

Shortly after they met, they married on December 15, 1935. Mama was 21 years old. They had a small apartment on the South Side of Chicago and Mama didn't work outside the home. Even after she married, she still helped her mother, preparing meals for her siblings and helping with the shopping. Once in a while she cleaned the houses on Dad's laundry route to make some extra money. It was a simple life of giving selflessly.

*Camille's First Holy Communion
with Mama and Dad (Rose and Anthony)*

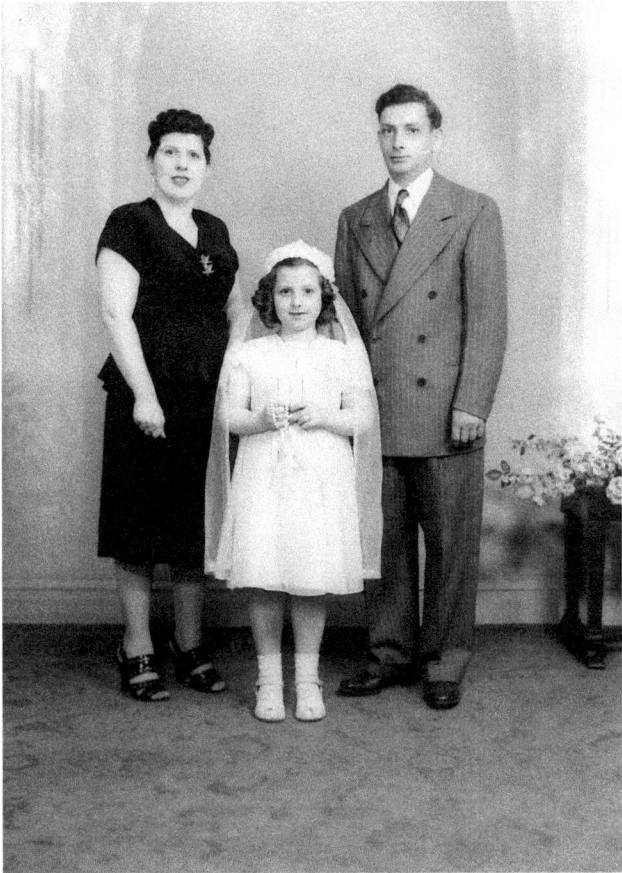

2

My Early Life

Mama and Dad had hoped for children, but it wasn't until five years later that I arrived. I was born at Mother Cabrini Hospital in Chicago on June 4th, one day before Mama's 26th birthday. I had lots of hair—Mama's curls and Dad's wavy hair. I was 12 pounds at birth and from then on an excellent eater. From the start, I was fed on pasta. I was a happy baby, so I am told, and well loved by my parents. Being a mother was Mama's most important and rewarding role, and she often told me that I was the light in my Dad's life. He was so proud of me that he couldn't find it in his heart to discipline me. All activities centered on the family. We spent Sundays at the park or on a picnic, or visited with family members after Mass. As a child, I liked that fact. I was always around adults and received lots of attention, for I was never quiet or shy. I had many uncles to make a fuss over me. My aunt and I were very close, too, because she was the youngest in Mama's family and the only other girl. Mama always said that even the dog at my grandma's house was very protective of me.

When World War II began, four of Mama's brothers joined the service. There was less work for the family, but Mama continued to help out at her parents' home even though most of her time was spent cleaning her own house, baking, and cooking. In her free time, she loved to spend time with her books. Mama read all she could about General MacArthur and the war and also collected pictures and articles about General Eisenhower. She even had a scrapbook of many of the articles written in the paper. When peace came, everyone was most grateful that all her brothers returned home safe from the service. After the boys came home, they made lives for themselves, married, and moved out of the house.

As time went on, we were at Grandma's house a great deal more because she was increasingly ill. When she died a few years later, Mama Rose brought her father and a single brother to live with us. We left our little apartment in the old neighborhood around Sangamon and Taylor and moved to a house on the West Side of Chicago. It was a two-flat, and one of her married brothers moved in upstairs. Again, the family was close together.

Life went on happily. Dad eventually did purchase a television. Mama still loved her books, her radio programs, and her Cubs games. She helped out at our church, St. Finbarr, and at the parish school which I attended from kindergarten to eighth grade. There were many parish and school fundraisers, and Mama always ran the bake sales.

Mama made sure I had a wonderful education. She had chosen a Catholic school for me because it had many good teachers who were Sisters of Mercy working in active ministry after taking simple vows. Having always loved school, I really enjoyed being with the sisters. I often stayed after school to help them. I even worked in the sacristy. On Fridays I used to go shopping with the sisters and carry their groceries. Inspired by their example, I decided very early in life that I wanted to be a teacher.

Special religious ceremonies like First Communions and Confirmations were big events for all in the family. There would be lots of folks, lots of laughter, and always lots of delicious food. Looking back, I remember how I looked forward to my First Holy Communion and all the celebrations that were planned. Receiving the Eucharist, the Body and Blood of Jesus, is a very special day for all Catholic children and I was very excited when my day came. As I look back, I am so happy that I had my Dad Anthony and Mama Rose with me at my First Holy Communion, because in a few months, our life as we knew it would change forever.

Camille and Mama Rose at church

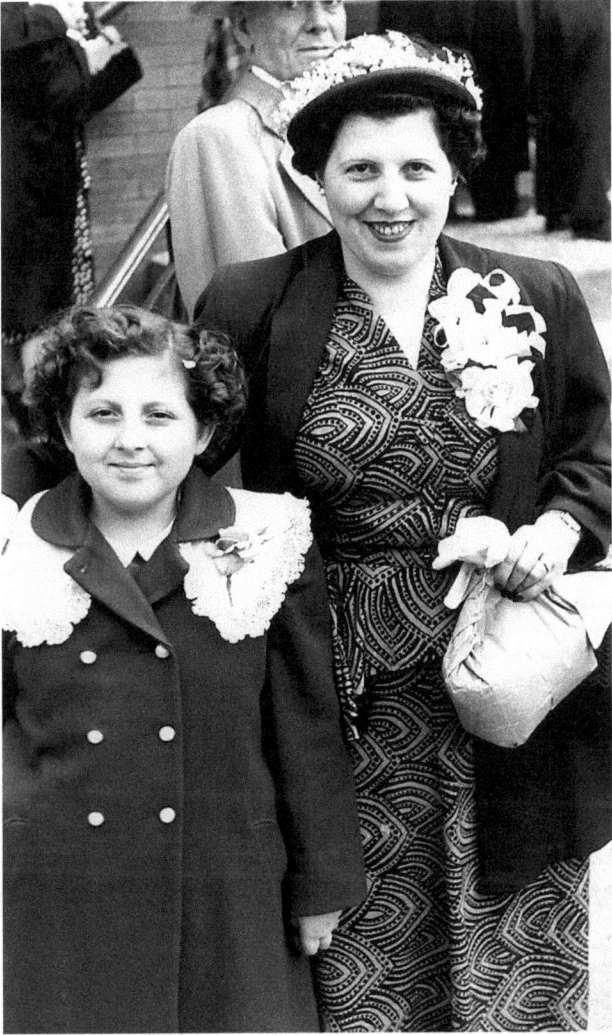

Mama Rose working at Motorola

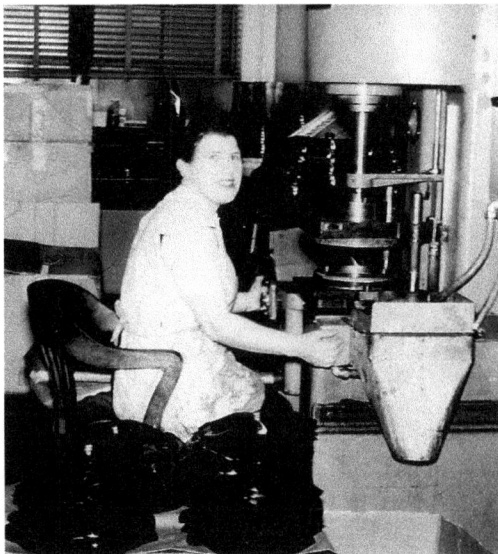

3

Life Without Dad

Suddenly, and without warning, my Dad, Mama's husband of 13 years, died from a heart attack. He went to the basement to get the hose to wash his car and collapsed. As a child, I didn't realize the impact this would have on us. I have few memories of my Dad, for I was only eight years old at the time he died. After my Dad's death, without an education, Mama was forced to enter the workforce. She first found work in a box factory near her home. She then looked for a better paying job and eventually worked on a piecework basis in several corporations such as Zenith and Motorola. Since she never learned to drive and we couldn't have afforded a car even if she had, Mama had to work long hours on her feet and then take a bus home and walk several blocks from the bus. Not having an education made her life difficult and her resources very limited.

Mama was working from early morn to early evening, so my grandfather often walked me to school, which was five blocks from our house. After I graduated from eighth grade, we moved to Berwyn and St. Mary of

Celle Parish. Uncle Jerry and Grandpa still lived with us. Berwyn had no resemblance to the liveliness of the old neighborhood around Sangamon and Taylor, except that Mama's siblings were all there. Since Grandpa was with us, the family had big parties at our home, our family custom for the rest of his life. My fondest memories of him were when he would spend hours reading his old worn-out Italian prayer book. He still loved his wine but no longer made it. Uncle Jerry still lived with us and he never married. He worked as a truck driver and was always a lot of fun to be around. He helped Mama with family responsibilities and finances when he could, but he himself often needed Mama to help him out. In return he brought laughter to us all.

Mama was careful with her money. She would buy one item of furniture needed at a time. She didn't go on vacation or spend money on herself. Nevertheless, we always had a table of wonderful rich-smelling foods to share and enjoy. Holidays were especially filled with wonderful home-baked cakes and cookies. The main courses were homemade pasta and all the Italian specialties, with family around for the feast. Mama would prepare for days, cooking and baking, and this was a joy for her. If someone gave her a compliment on her meal, she beamed with delight. It was easy to make her happy.

I'm sure Mama had big dreams and hopes for her future, but she never voiced them or complained that they were not fulfilled. Mama never dominated a conversation and was always in the background. If she expressed an opinion that was not accepted, then it was dropped. She never fought with anyone. She never swore at anyone or really ever raised her voice in anger. I often thought she must feel she couldn't win any argument. If she was disappointed in something, one had to really pry to know what it was. These were wonderful qualities, but in many ways made her a prisoner in her own person. So many times I would have loved to see her let loose and speak her mind, but this was just not in her nature. Mama was a peacemaker. She wanted peace at any cost, even if she didn't agree with the demands made on her by others. I tried many times to get her to speak up but this made her so uncomfortable. She was a quiet, loving person, eager to please others. She was even very quiet about her fears when we talked heart to heart. Her sacrifices were done so quietly that they often went unnoticed. Later in life I finally was able to understand and appreciate the extent of her sacrifice and all that she gave to others in her life.

Mama seldom initiated anything funny but could enjoy and laugh at a funny situation. She often received unwanted advice and didn't defend herself. In many ways, I always thought she was other-directed, dependent on her family. She didn't use her own power to make her own decisions. Her life was simply defined by her commitment to family: doing everything together, from shopping, to going to church, to visiting other family members. Her sister did her hair, her brothers drove her everywhere. They all met for Sunday Mass. On summer nights, the siblings sat in the yard and feasted on cake and coffee. On winter nights, they gathered to watch TV and have goodies. They made plans together and were very interdependent. Life was simple and that was good.

Mama and I spent a lot of time together visiting family because that was so important to her. We did a lot of other things, too. Mama's delights were very simple, such as going to the park or to downtown Chicago. We occasionally went to the Chicago Theater for a stage performance. We saw Roy Rogers and Trigger as well as Gene Autry on the theater stage. We went to all the cowboy movies at our local movie theaters. We made trips to Wrigley Field, for Mama was an ardent Cubs fan. She also enjoyed an ice cream banana split afterwards at a local soda shop. Another love Mama had was the Ice Capades with Sonja Henie. We went every year to as many shows as we could. And of course, every Christmas we ate lunch under the big Christmas tree at Marshall Field's. Sometimes we just walked around the downtown area window-shopping, enjoying the L ride to and from and the view of the city. We shared many happy times on these trips.

Perhaps because she herself was unable to complete her schooling, Mama made sure that I received a good education. I always appreciated my education and knew the sacrifice Mama made so that I could go to a Catholic school. When I graduated from eighth grade and was ready for high school, Mama insisted that I attend a Catholic school. I chose Siena High School on the West Side of Chicago where the teachers were also members of the Sisters of Mercy, the same religious order that staffed my parish elementary school. Those were wonderful years of fun-filled life experiences. I was a people person, had lots of friends, and enjoyed going to parties and participating in extracurricular activities. However, in my sophomore year, I was in trouble for talking too much. The sister would sprinkle me with holy water and even asked Mama to come in to speak with her about my behavior. Mama was so embarrassed to be called into school by a sister. As I was leading her up the stairs to the sister's room, she was hitting me (gently) for causing this problem. Thankfully, she never had to come to the school again, but I can't say I talked any less.

After high school I felt the call to religious life. Mama was not surprised when I told her about my plans to enter the Sisters of Mercy. When I left for the convent, Mama found this most difficult, but her own religious beliefs would not have her interfere with my decision. Mama had a strong faith in and acceptance of God's will in her life, and this time was no exception, even though it was difficult. My being an only child made it an even bigger loss for her. All the trips and movies we shared would no longer be part of our life together. I'm sure there was much loneliness for Mama, but again, as in the past, she bore it silently. Mama came to visit every visiting Sunday with Uncle Jerry. She brought me wonderful Italian goodies, which I missed very much. Once she revealed her dislike of calling the Mother Superior "Mother." "After all," she said, "you have only one mother and that is me—Mama Rose." She wrote to me as often as she could, but very little that was personal. Mostly her letters just said that she wanted to make sure that I was happy. She never let on about the changes in her life.

I saw very little of the family when I was in the convent because I was not allowed to come home to share in all the celebrations. However, when the time came for me to take my vows, we were allowed to have a party with our family. But first I had to make an eight-day retreat, eight days of silence. During retreat, I was called to the Superior's office and told there was an important call from my Mama. With permission to break the retreat, I went to the phone. Mama wanted to know: "Do you want beef and chicken at your party?" I couldn't believe this: Mama, what a sweetheart! And how innocent. She was so proud and wanted the best celebration she could afford for me with all my favorite dishes. It turned out to be a grand party with tons of food and lots of people at the Como Inn.

When I began teaching, Mama was very proud of my work and told me to be good to the children and not to fail them. She didn't ask many questions about my life or what it involved. For her, it was enough that it was good. Mama was concerned for my safety when I was working on the West Side of Chicago. When I was at St. Malachy's School, violence broke out after Martin Luther King, Jr. was killed. Even though we were in full habits, we knew the danger of being on the streets. All of Madison Street in our neighborhood was in flames, and our school was closed for many days. Mama made very little comment about the danger but assured me of her many prayers.

It was at a later time that I came to know how worried Mama had been about my living in the city. On this occasion, Mama and I went to Park Ridge on the Northwest Side to see my friend Sister Judy Stojsavljevic. She had invited us to see their brand new convent, which was very modern and beautiful, at St. Paul of the Cross School where she was teaching. Mama was hitting me (gently) saying, "What have you done that you're in the inner city in poor convents?" That's how I came to know Mama was worried about where I was living. About ten years later, after I had left the convent, I did go to St. Paul of the Cross as the kindergarten teacher. I told Mama that I finally made it to Park Ridge; her comment was simply, "So good!"

As Mama aged, her life was less financially secure. She worked on an assembly line and could no longer do piecework. She took only one vacation with a fellow factory worker to Hawaii. She saved for this trip for years. While she shared some pictures with pride after her return, she never said much about her experiences.

Her hobbies remained the same: cooking, baking, reading, working crossword puzzles, and following her favorite team, the Chicago Cubs. She occasionally went to Wrigley Field with her brothers, but mostly she listened to the games on the radio. Many nights she went to bed wearing headphones so she could hear the final out of the game. She would always say, "I hope I don't die before the Cubs win a pennant!" She gave me a love for the game as well as a source of entertainment and, most important, something to share with her. Every letter written to me when I was in the convent gave me the Cubs standings, batting averages, and all the news on Ernie Banks. When I was teaching in the city I wrote to Ernie and asked him to visit my class. Unfortunately he never was able to come.

After twelve years, I returned home from the convent. Mama was happy to have me home; it was as if I had never left. I was her "baby" again. When Mama and I talked on the phone, I would end the conversation with "I love you," and she would respond, "Me too." She waited up for me at night and wanted me home with her most of the time. If I looked for an apartment, she was devastated and would say, "You belong here!" I knew how she felt having me home again, and I never found that apartment. Mama didn't like the nickname the Sisters of Mercy I lived with had given me: "Ange." The sisters often had nicknames for each other and they thought the name fit me. I liked it too, for not only did I think I looked more like an Ange than a Camille but it was also Mama's sister's name. But Mama would have no part of this. If someone called her home and asked for Ange, she'd say, "No one here by that name" and hang up! She'd say to me, "You were baptized Camille, period."

Several months after leaving the convent, I met the man who was to become my husband and left home to get married two years later. I could sense Mama had mixed emotions about my leaving and found it hard to express these feelings; nevertheless, she gave me all her support. Before the wedding, Mama made plans to have my fiancé Richard and my future in-laws over for dinner to get to know them better. It was the beautifully planned meal that she could do so well with lots of Italian food, rich with olive oil and sauces for this lovely celebration. Mama knew that my future father-in-law was German and assumed that one of Richard's parents must be Italian, so she proceeded to ask my future mother-in-law, "Mrs. Grafer, what part of Italy are you from?" Margaret Grafer's response was, "I'm not Italian!" Mama was so upset to learn this; she didn't even have American bread in the house! I reassured her that Richard's parents loved Italian food. We all were able to laugh and the celebration went on happily, and despite Mama's initial embarrassment, she and my husband's mom always liked each other very much.

Even when wedding plans were being made, Mama was again in the background, while other relatives had much to say about my plans. If I showed displeasure at their interference, Mama, the peacemaker, would ask me not to say anything but to bear with the situation. We were married at St. Mary of Celle, my parish church, and at our wedding reception, Mama was in the back of the room quietly observing the celebration and greeting the guests with smiles and hugs. She was happy in her own quiet way. After the wedding, Mama made sure that she showed her approval of my new life by inviting my husband and me for dinner every Sunday. She made her wonderful pasta dishes and Italian sweets and often invited other family members for dinner. She loved company and she loved setting a nice table of special foods.

*Richard and Camille
before they were married*

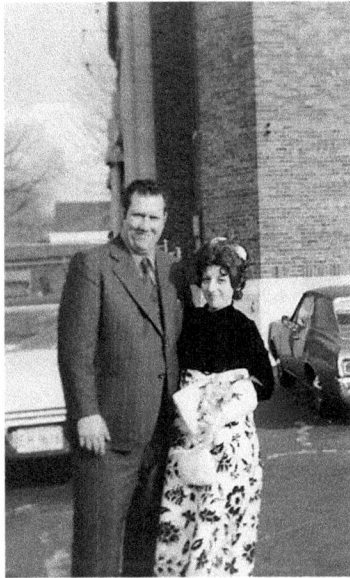

Margaret Grafer and Mama Rose

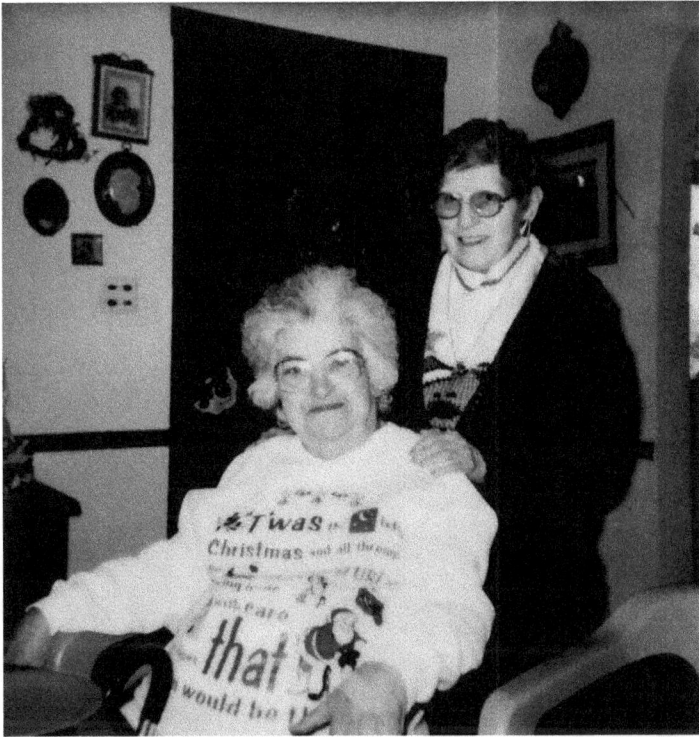

Mama Rose on Halloween

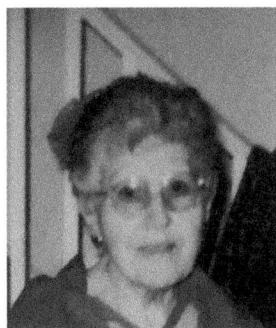

4

Seeing Changes in Mama

Mama as a rule was very healthy and very conscious of taking care of herself. Many illnesses came after she retired from working so hard for a long time. First, she had stomach problems. The doctor said it was brought on by the stresses she held inside. She suffered through congestive heart failure several times and each time she became a little more despondent. She was often in the emergency room with the same diagnosis: stress. I felt I needed to be more helpful and many times tried to get her to come live with me, but there was no way she would leave her home or her brother Jerry, who still lived with her.

Mama suffered through more tragedy in her later years. When her brother had a lung removed and needed a lot of attending to, she was the caregiver. And as a total shock, her only sister Angie had cancer of the eye and the eye had to be removed. Mama was there once again as a caregiver, helping her sister any way she could until my aunt finally lost her battle with cancer. This was difficult for all the family and especially for Mama because Angie was not only her sister but also her best friend. Even though Mama talked very little about her loss, I always felt her pain expressed through her sadness and tears.

She was great at caring for others, but not so good at taking care of herself. Mama was constantly feeling listless and out of sorts. She seemed to be failing fast physically. She read less and wasn't able to do her baking, which she loved. I had been faithfully going to her home every Sunday, but now that she was failing I was there from Friday to Sunday. In spite of all the medication she was on daily, I could see no improvement in her alertness. Finally, in spite of much disagreement from the family, I convinced Mama to try a new doctor. We were informed that Mama was over-medicated. Once her medicine was adjusted, she did gradually get better. Not terrific, but able to function with more regularity. She then went in for a hysterectomy at the age of 73.

All went well with the surgery, but afterwards I could see that her memory skills were failing. For several years her health had been very poor. Now she seemed to be more strong physically, quieter than ever, but more withdrawn, more confused. As time went on she became very "edgy" and began to be outspoken. She was frustrated with herself and with others. Suddenly she was beginning to lash out at her family and we were all in total surprise. I saw a change in her but I didn't think it was anything serious, probably because I was in denial. It was such a surprise to me when her brothers and sister-in-law took her to Rush-Presbyterian-St. Luke's Medical Center in Chicago for an extensive evaluation of her behavior. I had thought it was perhaps a good thing for her to finally emerge and be real in expressing her feelings. This new person seemed to be so liberated.

Mama Rose and Camille

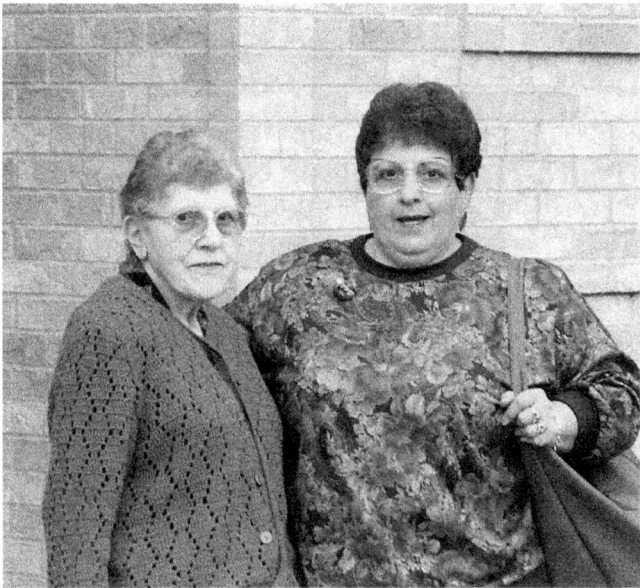

5

Accepting the Diagnosis

After the tests were concluded and evaluated, one doctor from the team at Rush–Presbyterian-St. Luke's met with us. We found out that Mama had Alzheimer's disease. This was in January of 1988. My first thought was disbelief since there was no history of this disease in the family. I had seen some changes in her, but I couldn't have predicted what the diagnosis would be. I had no knowledge of this disease or its effect on a person. The doctors were very clear in explaining Alzheimer's to us. Immediately I knew it would be a long road ahead for us because at that time there was no medication to cure it or to slow its progression. However, as the doctor spoke, I realized that her siblings were in denial; they didn't seem to understand what was being said to them. They repeatedly asked, "Is she doing these things on purpose?" I knew she would never be deliberately hurtful. I also realized that if Mama's brothers didn't understand the disease, then their responses could be detrimental to Mama's welfare.

This was a cruel realization: how uncomfortable people can be with someone who has the disease. The family had always been very vocal in Mama's life, so much so that lots of Mama's opinions or thoughts were not known to me. But now I knew that family would no longer be in the picture. It was evident that it was going to be just the two of us making life go on. I knew that I would have to and wanted to care for her to the best of my ability, even though I was not really able to visualize all that her care would involve. I understood that she would need guidance, but I was not sure what that would mean. This was a most difficult time. I did know, however, that I wanted to be sure that she would be as comfortable and safe as possible.

It is often thought that those suffering from Alzheimer's won't know if you are around. But your presence is so important. They are still people with feelings and are sad because they feel a loss of belonging. I always felt Mama was aware of the present moment.

While we were meeting with the lead physician in Mama's case, Mama was in the outer office with the receptionist. Suddenly the door to the office was flung open and Mama very loudly said, "What's taking you guys so long? I'm hungry and I want to eat!" I laughed and it was a moment of awakening for me, a light bulb moment. The former quiet and docile Mama would have sat in that outer office and waited, however long it took, without saying a word, even if she were hungry. This new Mama was very outspoken and expressed her feelings. After the meeting with the doctors, we went out to eat at a very nice Italian restaurant. Mama always ate very well and enjoyed pasta of any kind. I asked Mama if she enjoyed her cheese ravioli. She looked puzzled and replied, "Ravioli, what's that?" I was really surprised: This woman not only loved this delicious entrée, but had made ravioli herself for years. This was another light bulb moment for me.

When you are faced with the diagnosis of Alzheimer's for a loved one, it is likely that you will be overwhelmed by conflicting emotions: shock, denial, disbelief, grief, anger, guilt as well as love, stress as well as compassion, fear as well as understanding. We are never fully prepared for a tragedy affecting a loved one and especially for a tragedy which involves a parent's mortality. You will experience feelings surrounding the actions you take as well as the ones avoided. Don't be surprised or ashamed if some of these feelings arise in you as you try to cope and discover that you not only have to make decisions for your loved one but also to accept both the praise and criticism you will receive as a result. The decisions you will now have to make are based on your loved one's needs, your situation, and your religious beliefs.

Many mixed emotions were beginning to fill my head. Exactly where would all of this lead? There was a great deal of information given to all of us at this initial meeting with the doctor. It was all too much to absorb. I did realize, however, that I wanted Mama to live with me now that I knew this was something long-term. This illness would not lead to any improved situation, but rather deterioration. So while we believe one should be in control of one's life to maintain dignity, I knew that I would have to make decisions for Mama's future. I knew in my heart it would now be my time to be the caregiver, and that this was God's work for me now. Mama's siblings were not in agreement. They were frustrated with her outbursts toward them and couldn't cope with Mama's confusion or her raving shouts of anger, at them or at anyone who would listen. She was beginning to shout obscenities and tell everyone to leave her alone. Some of her outbursts were about her negative feelings about events in the past, feelings which perhaps had been building up for years. Suddenly, she was saying things she had held inside for so long. She not only knew the swear words she was using but also knew how to put them in context. Everyone was surprised when she would let loose with this assertiveness of power.

Shortly after the meeting, Mama's siblings called to ask me if we could put her in a nursing home. Since my year of teaching would end in just a few months and I'd be home for the summer, I asked them to give me a few weeks and I would move Mama to my home. The nursing home was not yet an option for me at this time. They agreed reluctantly to this arrangement and I began to make preparations.

Mama Rose and the first Duke

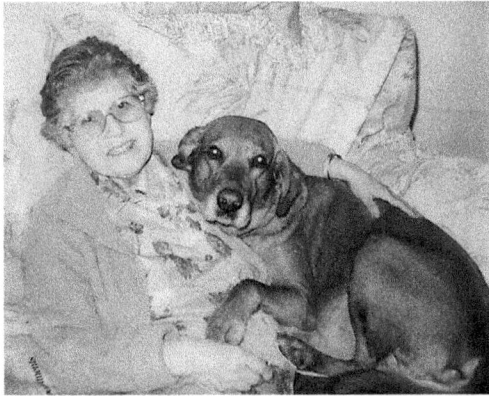

6

Settling Mama into My Home

In June of 1988, I started preparing to move Mama into the home I share with my husband Richard. I was hoping that I would be able to manage. I knew that I would be with her constantly and my life would be hectic, but my other responsibilities during the summer were not enormous. I did work full time but didn't have a family of children to come home to with their schedules and agendas. I thought of some of the caregivers I had met who had small children and full time jobs; for them, caring for a family member with Alzheimer's disease could be a tremendous burden.

But at that time, I began to look at the situation in a different way: I was afraid that the decision I had made would add to Mama's distress. In addition to her mental confusion, I was now going to expose her to new surroundings. I knew it was best to keep loved ones in familiar surroundings at their own home, but I could not do that. I was married and had to continue to work. Her single brother was still living at Mama's place, and I felt I really had no other choice but to bring her to my home. If she were healthy, I never would have been able to get her out of her own home, for I had tried many times before. But I had no choice. I moved all her bedroom furnishings and as much as I could of her most precious and personal items so that she would feel safe and somewhat comfortable with my husband and me. Actually, the transition was easier than I had thought it would be, because Mama was seemingly out of touch with reality. However, from day one I heard, "This is not my house. I want to go home." I felt guilty and sad thinking about how I would feel if I were uprooted from my independence, my home.

For a long time, I thought she meant her home in Berwyn, Illinois, but when I took her to Berwyn to visit, she had no recollection that this had been her home, nor did she recognize the house or the street. Surprisingly, when we visited St. Mary of Celle, the church she had attended for forty years, she told me, "Make a wish when you enter a new church." I was amused to hear this but it was helpful to know that some things, like making a wish, were not forgotten. I was still confused because it was a challenge to know exactly what she was trying to say when she would ask to go home. A long time later I came to realize that "home" was with God, for she would often say, "Why doesn't God want me?" Her looking forward to heaven was hard for me to understand until I realized that in reality, she was losing language and so she was expressing a feeling of longing, of wanting this, her current life, to end.

Mama was very pleasant most of the time. I tried to help her lead a life that was as normal as possible. I continued to take her to church even when Mama would talk out loud at Mass. I would take her to the "Cry Room" of St. Stephen's Church in Des Plaines near my home. She was louder than the children in that room. It was evident that this was not working for me or for her. Then I would let some time pass and try going to Mass again with Mama. Sometimes she was most respectful, but at other times she would let loose, talking or swearing.

Of course, there were many places she did not recognize on a daily basis. She wasn't sure why she was in a grocery store or in the hair salon. I often had to explain why we were in a certain place and what the task was at hand and reinforce this message several times.

Then there were people she no longer remembered. The hardest fact for me to realize was that she no longer knew me as her daughter although she always recognized me with a smile as someone who cared for her. I'd ask her, "Who am I?" and she'd laugh and say "Are you my friend? Are you my neighbor? Are you Mrs. X? Great!" And I'd give her a big kiss and hug and say "I love you," and her "I love you" came back to me loud and clear. Mama in her own way was displaying humor as well as affection and gratitude for her care.

> Be prepared that an open-ended question you ask such as "Who am I?" could lead to your having hurt feelings, but you have to learn to control them. The disease quietly consumes your loved one. The scrapbook of the past and all the memories of life fade into a blur. At this phase of the disease, your loved one still recognizes that something is wrong but doesn't understand the cause.

I am very grateful for the help I received at this time. My friend TC (Mary Therese Pallasch) referred me to Sister Lois M. Rossi, a Franciscan Sister of Chicago, who had worked in a nursing home and also taught classes in Licensed Practical Nursing. She had experience with people with Alzheimer's at all stages of the disease and was able to advise me and help me understand what was going on with Mama. She also made it very clear, as did my other friends, that I had to take some time for myself.

Through the years, I learned to nod or smile when I didn't know what Mama was trying to say. It was this new lack of verbal skills that could be baffling. If I laughed at Mama's incongruities, she laughed with me and wasn't embarrassed. If I got annoyed or kept throwing questions at her, she got angry and frustrated too—and the anger might last a long time. So I mostly chose to laugh rather than to be angry or hurt. Comedian Jay Leno once said. "You can't stay mad at someone who makes you laugh." Mama had her moments of frustration and I had mine. We made lots of mistakes, but we laughed a lot together. While her ability to understand words decreased, her sensitivity to emotions increased. Laughing with Mama was my way of coping with the situation.

While I tried to maintain a normal life for her, what was normal now? She had been a homemaker, a caregiver, an active person, and now she needed constant supervision. She was no longer independent, but I needed to make every effort to make her feel as independent as possible. The ease of her being able to perform basic tasks helped me establish the routine for both me and Mama. If I helped her dress and she chose to put something on backwards, I needed to ease her out of the clothes in a sensitive manner without showing frustration. I also found that what worked one day in getting her dressed did not work the next day. At times Mama was creative in the area of dressing. I never knew what she'd be wearing when she came down from her bedroom or if she would even be fully dressed.

During the day I tried to make Mama feel useful and worthwhile while maintaining her own dignity. This was my daily challenge: what to do daily, how much to demonstrate, how much to push, and how laid back to be. Should I take the clues from her or lead the way? This was a trial and error time for me. I often saw Mama get very stubborn about my plans and, rather than cross her, I kept coming up with new ideas. Always the question: What to do today? Let's try the kitchen. I thought she'd be most comfortable there. Mama had been a fabulous cook, but now, she couldn't initiate baking anything at all although she could still follow some directions. At times I wasn't sure she knew what we were trying to make for dinner. She still loved to eat and that would motivate her to help. I would help her stir something or follow through with some other simple task. We had to take everything step by step because Mama could no longer process the entire task. When a particular dish was finished, we always raved about what a good cook and baker she was and how well everything had been prepared. This made Mama beam with pride. Mama had always taken pride in her baking, even having recipes published in the local paper. I would now see her reading the paper and it would be upside down. Still, she would ask for the daily paper to check out the news and recipes.

All of her life Mama loved to walk, and she still did. When we didn't have any errands outside the home, she constantly walked in the house up and down the stairs with ease. I tried to take her out every day because she used to love to be out in the world and I hoped this would make her feel as normal as possible. We'd ride in the car, shop (or actually just walk around the stores), visit people, and stop in church. However, after a while she became uncomfortable and even refused to get out of the car. I had thought these outings would be fun for her, but most times it became frustrating and frightening since everything was unknown. Even when we were visiting friends, she often gave me the hardest time. We were invited to lunch at the home of one of the teachers and I of course took Mama. "Not getting out of the car," she said. I finally coaxed her out and we had a nice lunch with my colleague Pat Gill. Usually, Mama would respond better to other folks than to me, so when I was lucky enough to find someone else to help me, she'd cooperate. I had to remember not to let feelings get in the way but just get the situation settled: She's out of the car.

On another occasion, Richard and I had a friend's wedding to attend and I brought Mama. It was a late Saturday evening Mass and I brought my friend Mary Kay Hastings to care for her. Mama was cooperative with everyone most of the time, but sometimes she was not cooperative with anyone. I thought Mama would enjoy the wedding Mass. Wrong! Not a good idea. Mama was uncooperative if she was tired or if it was dark outside and this evening was no exception. She began talking out loud, telling the priest to speak up. Mary Kay had to take her out of church, but you could hear Mama talking all the way out. The guests at the wedding thought some kids were acting out. No, it wasn't children, but Mama Rose!

I found that the people we met when we were out were most understanding and wonderful with her when I told them she had Alzheimer's. They showed tolerance as well as understanding, for it seemed that everyone knew someone with the condition. Even if they were not knowledgeable about the disease, they could sympathize with her innocence and behavior. Many would just smile at her. When I took her grocery shopping, she would pick up batteries or any object around and fill the cart. Many a time she'd help herself to grapes or a banana. I remember one occasion when she was eating candy. Now Mama loved her chocolate candy bars such as Hershey Almond Bars and Milky Way. I thought she had taken it off the shelf of Kmart, but after I made her put it back, I saw the Easter Bunny giving out candy to all the children in the store. He must have seen the little child in Mama and her need for some candy, too. Once when we were at Dominick's, there was a long line for the checkout, so I sat Mama down on a bench and asked her to wait for me. Knowing that if she had something to eat she would stay in one place, I asked the checkout girl to give her a candy bar and I would pay for it when I purchased my groceries. When it was finally time to leave I said, "Come on Mama, let's go." "No, I have to wait for Camille," she replied (the checkout person who handed her the candy bar must be Camille!). "I'm Camille!" "No, you are not!" was her constant reply. The man sitting next to her gave her a funny puzzled look. He then realized what I was trying to do and made a friendly gesture to me and said, "Hi Camille!" Mama smiled, "Oh, you're Camille," and away we went laughing.

When my friend TC called Mama each day, she was thrilled. Every call had the same dialogue: "How are the kids?" "How's school?" Mama would giggle and tell me it was TC on the phone. Maybe she didn't remember the call afterward, but at that moment she was happy someone had called her. For a long time she was able to converse and carry on a conversation. Eventually she did get to the point where she wasn't aware of the phone or its function, but just for those moments of recognition when she did enjoy having a friend call, it was worth the fuss.

Mama would watch The CatholicTV Network. One program she loved was Mother Angelica. Mama would always say, "That nun is very happy." She would laugh

with her even if she didn't realize why she was laughing. The Mass was on television three times daily and she
would watch it over and over, not remembering that she
had just seen the same Mass. Mama and I were also able
to say the Rosary since the prayers are repeated and easy
to remember. She was also able to say it along with a program on this Catholic channel. She remembered songs
and prayers she had learned in the past; they definitely
stayed in her memory. She found much comfort in relat-
ing to God because her faith had been such an important
part of her life before the disease, and it still was.

In many ways, Mama was free from all the pressures
of life because she didn't set her own agenda anymore.
She had no more worries about money, bills, or obliga-
tions. She would have some moments of reflection, however. Some of her behaviors were foreign even to her and
she would have a concerned look on her face, as if to
ask, What's going on? Often she would ask me, "What
is wrong with me?" We never really gave Mama an explanation of her disease and how it was affecting her
behavior since we had difficulty digesting all of the im-
plications ourselves. She was beyond understanding this
disease. When she was questioning her own behavior, I
became accustomed to telling her that she was fine and
not to worry.

One of the really special times in Mama's life at this
time was her attachment to our dog Duke. Growing up
as a child, I had wanted a dog but we never had one because Mama didn't want the hassle. My Dad had brought
a puppy home one day and it was gone the next. It had
cried all night and made a mess on the floor. Now that
Mama was living with us, she wanted our Duke with her
at all times. She loved Duke and Duke loved her. He was
a large dog but very patient and well-behaved. We had

posted a sign, "Beware of Dog," but any time we were home or had company, Dukie had a pink ball in his mouth ready to play. Mama talked to him all day and threw his ball over and over. She played "This little piggy went to market. . ." on his paws. She spent most of each day with Duke (and if Duke had enough of Mama Rose, he'd hide in the closet upstairs). He would sit next to her on the couch for hours and Mama found it easier to talk to the dog than to anyone else. I often got a kick out of her conversations with him. Mama sang repeatedly, "God loves me and God loves Dukie too." And her favorite song, "You Are My Sunshine," was often sung to Dukie. If the dog came near my husband or me, she would get jealous, call him to her side and say, "Dukie, you don't love me anymore?" Mama always fed him part of anything she was eating. He often wore food if she missed his mouth. One day when we were saying the Rosary together, she told Duke to pray with us. My reply was. "He can't talk, Mama!" Her answer to that was "Yeah, well he talks when he wants to!"

Mama and I needed to find moments to cherish and make wonderful memories at this time in our lives, moments when we connected. There was never any doubt about the love between us. There were lots of hugs and kisses between us. The connection we found was laughter and little talks. There was a one-liner here and there that would end in laughter and enjoyment and we made sure there was plenty of this on a daily basis. Mama got to the point where she always had a comeback line that I thought was hysterical. Keeping Mama in a pleasant mood made it a lot easier for me as well as for others to be around her too. Some people did not know what to do or how to respond to her, but our laughter made them relax. Some thought our laughter was disrespectful and they were uncomfortable with it. They thought we were making a joke out of a very sad disease. However, humor carried Mama and me through a difficult journey. One day she made me laugh when she said, "Camille, you should be a teacher, you always wanted to be a teacher." "Mama, I am a teacher and have been for many years." She smiled and said, "Wow, that's good."

The second connection we found was singing together. When I was a teenager there was a television program called *The Hit Parade* and we watched it faithfully. We also had bought records of all the popular songs that were published and we sang together for hours. Mama still remembered words to the "oldies" and she got a kick out of this. We would spend hours singing songs like "Daisy," "Let Me Call You Sweetheart," and the like. She loved "You Are My Sunshine" the best and we sang it at the beginning, middle, and end of our singing sessions. Music always lifted our spirits. I often heard Mama singing to Dukie, "Sing Dukie, sing with me!" and then she would continue singing. Duke just sat there, loving the attention. At times I could also get Mama to dance with me. She would giggle with delight. Then Duke would pounce around too, and again, the giggles.

My husband worked for the Forest Preserve District and we rented a house in the heart of the forest when Mama was living with us. Mama loved the grounds but thought it strange we had no neighbors other than the animals. The deer would come right up to our windows because we had a salt block out for them. Once when a deer ran by us on the road around the house, Mama commented, "My, that's a big dog." We were careful to check the dogs often for deer ticks. Once Richard discovered a tick in Mama's arm and wasn't able to remove it for it was very deep, so we headed to the emergency room to have it removed. She never complained of having pain and thank God didn't realize the danger of a deer tick bite. The doctors thought she would have no reactions from the tick, but we watched her closely anyway with thankful prayers when she showed no symptoms.

Summertime provided a relaxed time for making many good memories. Mama had a terrific warm smile that made everyone around her happy. We had many laughs as well as some tears. I now look back and cherish even the difficult times when I was frustrated. This new Mama Rose often made us laugh and she often laughed at herself. There was less pressure on her to try to figure out what was happening to her abilities and more freedom from having to please others. She was showing more and more independence. As the summer progressed, however, I saw changes in Mama. She was not as quiet as before and she seemed more aggressive. She stood her ground and if she didn't want to do something, she didn't do it. At times we would avoid a problem by letting her choose what to do, like dressing in some outrageous combination of clothing for the sake of expressing her independence.

Along with Mama's sense of humor came a lot of swearing that was NEVER in her vocabulary, but appeared to be stored in her brain. One of her caregivers said Mama sounded like a foul-mouthed lumberjack. She had these swear words in and out of context for everyone in sight. This not only had me stunned, but laughing. It was so out of character! She also had many moments of frustration and anger that were horrible. There were hours of her being aware of everything but behaving out of control. I recall weekends when she screamed and raged for well over 24 hours. No one and nothing could settle her down. During these bouts, I would stay up with her and wonder where she found the stamina to keep going. Those hours of screaming and anger really hurt me, for I realized there was a deep agony inside. Some frustration or awareness of her inability to control a situation must have triggered this extreme behavior. It was difficult to know how to help her so I let it run its course. After the rage was over, she would sleep deeply for hours.

A person with Alzheimer's may express feelings in the form of rage because they cannot articulate a problem. Do not be upset if hurtful words are directed at you. Remember that it is the illness talking, not the person you knew.

During these times of rage, Mama would tell me that I was no good, not even as a child, always trouble. I could laugh because I knew it was her illness causing her to say such things. I learned to ignore the remarks and go on, making humor out of it if I could. To get angry with her for something she couldn't help was no benefit to anyone. Mama also made use of many defense mechanisms and did not take responsibility when something went wrong. Her favorites were "Do it yourself" and "I didn't do it!" She blamed the dog for many things that dogs can't do. In this way, Mama was maintaining some dignity by her quick defense. We recognized her fight and just let things go.

Long nights are very exhausting to anyone, especially the caregiver, because what the night will bring is an unknown. Even though I was a night person, I had to get enough sleep. It was often difficult to go to bed early, especially if Mama wasn't sleeping. Her evenings were often very "busy" and sleep was often broken up for her and for me. Even when Mama was sleeping, I felt I needed to be aware and ready in case she woke up suddenly.

One night she woke me up to help her put on her earrings. We laughed because they were M&Ms and I suggested she just eat them instead. On another occasion Mama came to my room after my husband left for work because I was sleeping in, so I told her to get in the bed with me. No sooner was she in bed than she started to talk: "I love God, God loves me." She repeated this many times. So I repeated many times, "No talking. Time for sleeping!" There was a pause and then I heard her again, "I love God, God loves me and you're a b----." I laughed so hard I shook the bed. Then I heard her say laughingly, "Oh you laugh at everything, everything is funny to you, go to sleep." I heard her giggle as the bed shook again. Yet another time I was awakened by Mama's faint cry for help. Running to her room and not finding her there had me in a panic. After searching the house, I realized she was in her bedroom closet. She had gone in and somehow the door closed behind her, and she was baffled and did not know how to get out of there. I told her this was no time for hide and seek and led her back to her bed.

My Bunco group, who always gave me their support,
welcoming Mama to our Halloween party

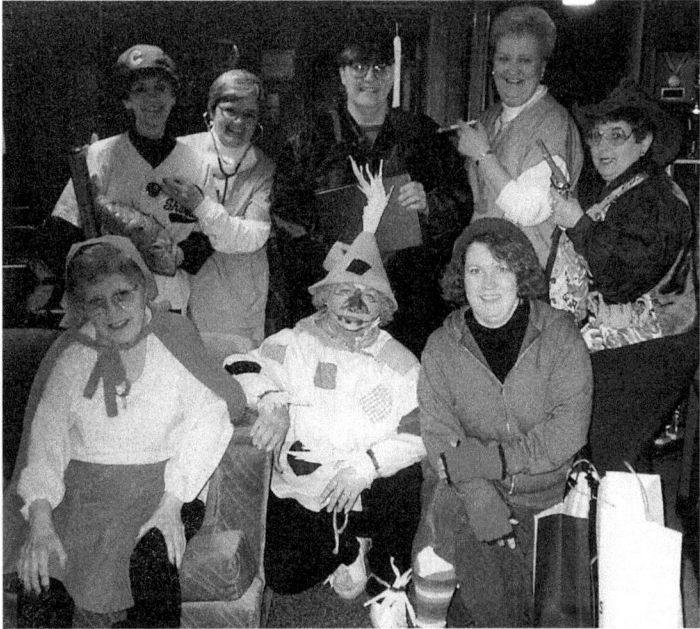

7

Searching for a Caregiver

As the summer was ending and the new school year beginning, we were entering a new stage because now it was necessary for me to find a caregiver who could care for Mama while I was at work. Care requires a lot of patience, kindness, and understanding, and of course, a knowledge of the disease in all its aspects. Until this point, I really hadn't looked beyond the initial stage of caregiving, but went from day to day. There seemed to be no need. Mama could be out of sight in her bedroom, she still could be left alone in the yard, and she was dressing herself and able to do some chores around the house. Looking back, I see now that I should have been more prepared for all the stages to follow and in touch with the options available to me for acquiring the best care for Mama.

As we began this new phase, I was beginning to see drastic contrasts in Mama's behavior. I really did a great deal of learning. I found myself constantly problem solving. Mama and I were both learning new roles and I had to learn how to eliminate her frustrations as best I could and assure her that I understood her needs. She needed more hands-on help with eating and dressing and she had to be watched more carefully so she wouldn't get hurt. I read a great deal about the disease but I didn't consult with anyone who had gone through the same experience.

Even though I knew I could get information and support from a group, I just felt it was too much of a burden for me to attend these sessions. I would be teaching, needed a lot of time for class preparation, and couldn't attend a meeting unless I found a caregiver for Mama even for that short time.

Many folks find support groups to be very enlightening and helpful. Often you can get in touch with an Alzheimer's Support Group in your area through your local community center or hospital. These groups will be able to give you information about resources that are available to the elderly and helpful suggestions about reaching out to the person with Alzheimer's. It's also good to share your feelings in a group that is experiencing the same situation and to learn that you are not alone in dealing with the care of your loved one.

I did find I needed a break more often and had to ask for help so I could get things done in my home. My strongest support came from my friends who were so wonderful, helping me and reaching out to Mama throughout her illness. I appreciated their kindnesses so much and will always be grateful. I was able to share my experiences daily with them because they truly enjoyed "Mama Rose" stories. At times these stories became my main conversation piece as I shared the funny situations and difficult times I encountered. I tried not to be a burden or to be limited in my conversations with others, but one can easily become consumed with the situation. I was also very grateful that I was working full time and was able to be involved in my work, which allowed me to be in a different environment with different folks. I was also fortunate to be teaching little ones in kindergarten, who lift your spirit and offer lots of laughter and hugs of love. The children always renewed my spirit.

I also needed time alone. I needed to be alone to shop, to pray, to read, and to rest. When could I fit all this in a day or a week? That was my first question. Sometimes it was difficult to prioritize my life. Finding time for reading was a challenge, but I needed to focus on something other than my care for Mama. When I found time to reflect rather than clean the house, I found I was coping better. The caregiver can easily drive herself to emotional exhaustion so I also made every effort to keep my attitude on track. If I saw the time with Mama as a burden, then she would become aware of my feelings. Unfortunately, we learn from our mistakes, but when there were times it was difficult to laugh, I prayed for patience and fought off the negative feelings. I focused on the fact that we didn't know how much time we would have together. Mama Rose's precious innocent nature made each day a new one. We were forming marvelous memories and I needed those to be genuine.

Mama's care also meant that my husband and I found our lives changed. We had to make time for each other to talk, have dinner, or see a movie. We didn't go out socially very often because we would have to leave Mama alone and I always had to ask my friends to stay with her. Most times we took Mama with us if we were sure she would enjoy the trip.

Physicians and counselors advise a caregiver to have some time alone, away from their loved one. Even when you feel you are doing your best, you are searching for ways to bring more quality into the Alzheimer person's life. This means not only that you must have lots of energy but you have to maintain a positive attitude as well. Be sure to make time for yourself without feeling any guilt. Stay connected to your friends, your interests, your faith, and your hobbies, and above all take good care of your health.

Care can be very expensive and often caregivers are afraid to be responsible when they know the person has Alzheimer's. First, I had to look into Mama's financial situation in order to plan carefully. In going through many sources of information, I learned that Mama was eligible for aid from the State of Illinois which would provide three hours of care per day as well as some financial support. Since I needed someone for eight hours and not three, the added time would have to be funded by Mama's Social Security and pension as well as my own money. There was never a question of whether I would do this or not. I was committed to giving her the care she needed. But I noted that this financial cost was not tax deductible, and funds are not available for home care. This can be a terrible burden for families facing Alzheimer's.

I met with a social worker recommended by my own physician and paid by Medicare and then began to look into home health care agencies and what they had to offer. I was very worried when it came to hiring a caregiver. So often one hears of abuse and a lack of tenderness toward the elderly. But I had no choice: I had to return to work and therefore was at the mercy of a social worker and under the pressure of time. And if I were at work and not able to supervise the caregiver, I felt I was at her mercy too. I hoped during all the hours I was away from home that Mama was not in a dangerous situation.

While the state would provide a caregiver, one problem is that the state's pay scale is appalling. Another problem is that their caregiver training for Alzheimer's disease is extremely limited. State-assigned helpers are basically trained to come in, clean house, and shop. They are knowledgeable in doing some limited tasks for the patient, like giving a bath, combing hair, and helping with dressing, but prefer not to do these things. In addition, the state had difficulty finding someone for us because the caregiver would have to drive to our home near Barrington in the forest preserve. There was no public transportation that was accessible from the train. This limited the number of workers the state could assign to us because few workers had their own transportation.

I employed several state workers who did not work out. The first person assigned to us was cleaning my house and helping herself to its contents, none of which I missed until I went to look for something and found the item gone. Despite the stage of her illness, Mama related some information to me about this caregiver, constantly telling me, "She doesn't talk to me." Communication with Mama was difficult and it was clear to me that this worker didn't know anything about Mama, nor did she want to know. Once I discovered the motive behind her housecleaning, I chose to let her go.

The second person from the state was a nice woman who was homeless and living out of her car. In her subtle way she hinted that she wanted to sleep at my house. She asked to sleep in our driveway, but we were living in the forest preserve house rented from the county and therefore we couldn't allow her to stay. I would often offer supper but would have my husband ask her to leave for the evening because I found it difficult to ask her to do so. At first I felt terrible, even though I knew my husband and I needed time with each other. My evenings were also very full preparing lessons for the next day as well as doing things with Mama. This woman made us feel uncomfortable since it appeared that to her we seemed to have so many material things. Later I came to learn that she was also collecting state aid and did have a place to live. Finally, we decided to let her go. The fact that she had lied and was taking advantage of our kindness made me wonder what she was doing with Mama.

The third person assigned to us by the state had to bring her dog with her. She told us she was homeless. I did not make any offer to make her feel my home was her home. I probably was very rude this time around after the experience with the caregiver before her. The fact that she had a dog irritated Mama no end, because this was Duke's home and Mama did not take at all to this other little dog. Mama told me over and over, "Send that dog home." Mama also said that this woman watched TV all day. I don't know if that was true, but she really seemed to get on Mama's nerves. This caregiver was also not always clean or soft-spoken. When I would inquire about their day together, she reported very little that she and Mama had shared. This was a strong signal that perhaps nothing was going on between them. I chose to let her go shortly after her assignment with us.

The fourth person assigned to us by the state was in my home for a very short time. One day when I came home from school she told me she had a sore back and proceeded to tell me she found some of my husband's ointment. She had taken the liberty of going through our medicine cabinet and had Mama rub this ointment on her back. Well, she, too, was soon gone. This behavior was neither acceptable nor appropriate. Obviously, even though she was not our idea of a caregiver, I was grateful that she was honest in telling me what she had done because I wouldn't have received this information from Mama. Keep in mind that I was paying these caregivers very well in addition to what they received from the state so that they would be well compensated and make Mama's day meaningful. But it wasn't working out.

So we started the whole process again, all in one school year. There was so much time spent in screening and hiring these caregivers: the phone calls with the state supervisor, the paperwork, the interviews—it was all frustrating and time consuming. I decided I couldn't depend on the state for the kind of help I wanted for Mama. The social worker then suggested I myself work for the state, since Mama was entitled to three hours of paid services, and she told me how to register for training. I did so, and through my own experience I became aware of the limited training given state workers and the poor pay scale offered at that time. Of course, I still needed to find my own person to care for her for the rest of the time I'd be away, for the full eight hours while I was in school. Nevertheless, working for the state gave me an opportunity to hire desirable caregivers that I could trust to make Mama their number one priority. Let me mention that there is no sense or reason for the amount of paperwork involved in getting some necessary aid for the elderly. I filled out duplicate forms with our life histories. Then I repeated the whole block of information again on the phone, only to find I now needed to come in for an interview. Then there would be a social worker out to see us in our home in a few weeks. Through experience, I became aware of the apparent lack of communication between social workers and their supervisors. Perhaps this was the reason for all the forms and repeated information.

I regretted that I hadn't been knowledgeable about assistance for the elderly. The "system" doesn't make this information readily available. I sought lots of advice and guidance in this area. After more sessions with a social worker, I found out Mama was also eligible for food stamps. I filled out more forms and held more phone conversations. Then I found out Mama would receive only eight dollars a month, which would only take care of her monthly orange juice supply but nothing else. I was grateful for the aid, but something seemed wrong here. I investigated further and after filling out more forms and talking to more social workers, I learned that Mama was eligible for at least twenty-five dollars a month.

The school year was over and now I was working for the state. I was required to attend several meetings a year for training. These sessions were an eye opener for me. The training itself consisted only of videos or short papers to read with absolutely nothing on the practical level and no hands-on training. While the videos were being shown during the training sessions, some workers would talk or read and not pay attention. There wasn't a quiz or any reinforcement of what we saw or read. Many workers came in late, some carrying bags of all their belongings. A couple of times I asked the workers about their living arrangements and found many to be homeless. I also asked how they were able to get to the patient's home and learned they used public transportation that was included in their pay. I often asked the caregivers if they were knowledgeable about dementia and Alzheimer's disease and learned from hearing about all their experiences that they had limited knowledge of either condition. The pay scale was terrible. In 1990 I was earning $3.75 an hour and was eventually raised to $4.00 an hour as caregiver. Low pay and little training were the culprits to be blamed for the poor performances we experienced with the state-appointed caregivers we hired. After all, this is not a very attractive job or a lifetime career. Yet many of the caregivers were older women and men and had been doing this for a long time. The care of our elderly is so important and the services so limited. I hope conditions will be better now in the 21st century. I do know that the State of Illinois has recently improved the training requirements for caregivers who work with people with Alzheimer's, so perhaps the situation will improve.

Nicki, Mario, and Lauren Servedio,
whose mother Terri was a caregiver for Mama,
visiting on Mama Rose's birthday

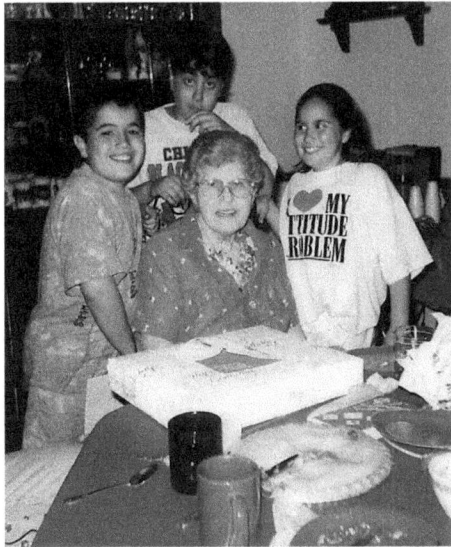

8

Finding In-home Care for Mama

After having explored the options given to me by the state, I had to look for a situation that would be more suitable to our needs. I needed to find a person I could trust to be with Mama while I was at work. I was quite sure Mama needed sociable surroundings and stimulation outside of the home. No matter how old one gets or how deteriorated one becomes, social interaction with other people is essential for good health, validating the person and making the person feel worthwhile. I was lucky to find that my niece through marriage was willing to help me out for a short time. Terri Servedio as caregiver finally provided me with peace of mind. She would drop her son Nicki off at school and then come over to my house to care for Mama. At this stage, Mama was able to stay home alone for the short time between my leaving and Terri's coming. Terri was terrific with Mama, and Mama liked her right away. This made a big difference in Mama's demeanor; she was happy. They would bake together, go out for lunch, shop, and visit with other folks. Mama was very agreeable and I was most pleased that finally we had a great arrangement. Terri would take Mama to pick up her son Nicki at school and then Nicki would spend time at our house too. Nicki was about eight years old and even at his young age, he enjoyed being with Mama, and she liked having a young person around. Nicki recalls that when the phone rang Mama would pull the plug of some appliance out of the wall and say "Hello." When no one spoke she replied, "Then the h--- with you!" Despite his young years, he realized that Alzheimer's was a terrible disease, but he really enjoyed being with Mama and said she was one funny lady. He laughed with Mama Rose and loved her.

It was summer again and I was home. Mama enjoyed sitting on the porch with our Duke. She also took walks with me through the forest preserve. We did some cooking, shopping, and lots of rides in the car, enjoying the beauty of the summer landscape. My friend TC took Mama for ice cream, which she always enjoyed. We would take her to the movies and when the popcorn was gone, we knew we soon would be leaving too because she would start to talk loudly and make it clear we had to be going home. June was time for Mama's birthday. My niece Rose Servedio and her children along with Terri and her family came to celebrate with us. Mama loved having young people around her. She got such a fit of giggles when we sang "Happy Birthday" to her, so naturally we sang it many times to see her happiness and hear her laughter. It was a grand party and one I remember for all the fun, the delicious good food, and the beautifully decorated cake that Terri made for Mama.

Mama touched a lot of lives and left good impressions with many people. This made my life easier when I needed time away. The manners she had learned in childhood stayed with her throughout the stages of her

90

disease. Mama always said "Please" and "Thank you" in all appropriate contexts. She was very appreciative and pleasant, so others were willing to stay with her and really did enjoy her company. Some of my closest friends were those who belonged to my group of friends who played Bunco (a game of dice rolling). Being able to take her with me to Bunco each month was great. Mama didn't understand the game, even though it is very simple, involving counting the numbers on the dice after each roll, but she enjoyed playing and being part of the group. If Mama had to roll the dice over and over she'd say, "I'm playing by myself," and giggle in delight. In spite of the fact that she didn't know what she was doing, she won all the time! The girls would be amazed. I would tell them, "She wins because she concentrates on the game and we're all laughing and talking!" The girls were wonderful, keeping her on track and seeing if she needed to roll again. The prize wasn't important; it was winning and the fuss we made over her that made her so happy. Mama couldn't enter into the conversation or all the laughing, but she laughed with us anyway. After much coffee and conversation, Mama would let me know it was time to head home. When it was my turn to host the group at my home, Terri helped Mama make pizza. The girls raved about the food and Mama beamed all night. As the years passed, it became more difficult for me to take her or have her stay to visit after the game, but the times we had at Bunco were wonderful memories.

It was about this time that our dog Duke won a weekend for four at the Pheasant Run Resort in St. Charles, Illinois (we put his name on the raffle ticket). TC and Mama and I had one room and my husband Richard had the other room. Mama was very comfortable with the trip. I was afraid she would find new surroundings frightening but all the people she knew were there and she must have felt safe. We all had a chance to walk the grounds, Richard swam and played some golf, and Mama watched us as we played cards. We had great room service that provided treats for Mama as part of our winning package as well as three fantastic meals served each day. Mama enjoyed eating every meal. The whole weekend ended beautifully providing a wonderful memory for all of us.

Even though the summers were less stressful for everyone, the summer of 1993 was very difficult because our beloved Duke was very ill. He was a beautiful Golden Retriever who loved to play constantly and was dearly loved by all of us. We had Duke to the vet several times that summer but they couldn't figure out what was wrong with him. To this day we don't know. We all were very sad, not only because he was so loved but also because he was Mama's friend and she was always with him. That last night, I stayed up with Duke, who was in pain. Richard and I knew we had to let him go peacefully. We couldn't have him suffering. Each dog you have is so special in its own way, but Duke was more than special; he was a life-saver for Mama. The decision to put him down was most difficult for us. Mama was sad when we told her Duke went to heaven, but I thought somehow this would be more devastating than it seemed. We knew she loved that dog so much, but actually, she couldn't show the emotion we thought she would. Richard and I were so afraid Mama would shut down in search for Duke, her buddy, so we immediately went in search of a puppy. The puppy we chose was a Chocolate Labrador and we named him Hershey. We even had the candy wrapper posted in several places so Mama would learn his name. No way. He was Duke to her. Most of the time he was Devil Dog! We learned that our idea of a replacement dog was not working and had been a mistake, for puppies do not sit still. He ran around, was into everything, and was too active to please Mama. This dog had Mama upset all the time. We had to give him away because Hershey raised her anxiety level. We tried several puppies, but none made Mama happy. Then we decided to advertise for an older dog . . . about two years old or more. It is harder to bond with older dogs, but they are usually calm and content to sit and would meet Mama's needs better than a puppy would. We were lucky that my sister-in-law, who always enjoyed Mama's company when she visited, realized we had to have a dog right away for Mama. She brought us a two-year-old dog that needed a home because the owner had died, and she thought that "Brooklyn" would be a good dog for Mama. "Brooklyn" was in the house for two seconds when Mama was calling him "Duke." So we had another Duke, and he was just plain Duke forever after that. All our dogs were Duke to Mama, and therefore to us.

The summer was coming to an end, and once again I had to make another major decision about Mama's care for the times when I would be teaching and away from her. I loved the wonderful country atmosphere of the big forest preserve house in Barrington, but it was really a hard place to reach with a car and nearly impossible without one. It was difficult to find someone I could trust to come out there to care for Mama. We still had our house in Des Plaines and I decided to move back. I hoped that it would be easier for me to find someone to care for Mama there. On the other hand, I was concerned that it was going to be another major move for Mama and I was afraid it would be traumatic. To my surprise she made the adjustment very easily because she liked seeing houses and folks passing by the front window. This house was more like a home for Mama.

There were some problems, however. Duke was forever running away from the yard. When the dog would run off in Barrington, it was all forest preserve land. Now in Des Plaines, I was concerned that the dog would be hit by a car or wouldn't know how to come back home. I was always concerned about losing Duke and having Mama so upset. She was always angry with me when Duke took off for his runaway stunt. He probably would have come back home on his own, but I couldn't take the chance. So I'd get in the car and chase that dog, often many blocks from home, until he was ready to come back. One day he ran down the street and I told Mama to watch for us in the window as I took the leash and went out to find him. As I came back toward the house, I saw Mama in the window. She had started to undress! Another time I had him on the leash, groceries in the other hand, and called Mama to follow us into the house. No way! She headed across the street. I had the challenge of losing Duke or losing Mama. It's a good thing I always told myself that I had to keep laughing. I put Duke in the house and then went to fetch Mama.

Mama had to do her thing. She would often disappear into her bedroom to rearrange things and to change clothes during the day, even though dressing and undressing was a challenge for her these days. When she reappeared, would she be fully dressed? One day I returned home from school to find Mama in what appeared to be a mini skirt! I knew she didn't own one. What she had done is to take a turtleneck sweater, tuck in the sleeves, and wear it around her waist. That was very creative, Mama!

In my search for a caregiver I contacted a social service agency in Park Ridge that helped seniors in the community. They were very compassionate and suggested a woman who lived close to my home in Des Plaines. She was older, very kind, and experienced with the illness since her own mom had shown signs of this disease and was now in a nursing home nearby. She was a good caregiver for Mama and we appreciated all she did. Our families even shared Thanksgiving. Unfortunately, Mama often gave her a hard time. As spring came, Mama refused to leave the house for the last two months of the school year. Soon it was June and summer again. I would be home with Mama full time, but we were losing our wonderful caregiver. She had some health problems of her own and would not be returning for the following autumn.

The summer was my time to be with Mama all day. She helped me around the house by folding towels or matching socks. They were all white so it made no difference how she did it. She also enjoyed some rides in the car with me on occasion. Being terrible with directions, I would often be going the wrong way. When I had to turn around in someone's driveway because I missed my street, she would say, "Made a mistake! Are you lost again?" She always giggled about my poor sense of direction. I'd say to her, "This you remember!" We could still enjoy a movie, shop, eat out, and even go to the concerts in the park in Park Ridge where she liked seeing all the people. She didn't like that I talked to everyone; she wanted my undivided attention. To keep Mama entertained, I had to have food, and when the food was gone it was time to move on. Also if it was getting dark, it was a signal that we had to head home.

I still was able to take Mama on fun outings. Everything had to be quick with Mama, so there was no sitting around after a meal or standing in line at the movie theater for tickets. When Mama was fine, we had a pleasant time. People seemed to recognize her anxiety and were very kind to accommodate us by moving us to the head of the line or helping in some other way. But when Mama was not agreeable, I found myself making excuses for her or trying to explain her condition. I wanted everyone to understand Mama but I also wanted to be fair and not impose on those who failed to see the dimensions of the disease. Generally, every outing with Mama was an opportunity to help others understand the condition and learn how to be compassionate toward those suffering from Alzheimer's.

Once, my friend Nancy Okerstrom and I had made plans to see a movie with our moms. Upon entering the theater, Nancy and her mom Anne got in line for popcorn. Mama was not going to wait; we had to go in quickly to get good seats. I told Nancy, "We'll go in and save your seats." So I sat Mama down and put two napkins on the seats between us to be saved for Nancy and Anne. A woman resembling me with the same color hair and about the same physical size sat down in front of Mama. Suddenly, Mama hit this lady on the head with her purse and said in a rather loud voice "You s-- -f a b----, why am I sitting here all by myself?" I said, "Mama, I'm over here next to you." The woman turned in anger, but when I quickly told her Mama had Alzheimer's disease she smiled and was very understanding about the situation. With an apology to this woman, we all laughed together. It was one of those outings that was filled with lots of surprises and many good laughs. After the movie (one we saw all the way through), we went for ice cream and Mama ordered a fudge sundae, which came with a rolled sugar cookie. She took the cookie out of the dish and said in a loud voice, "I never smoked and I'm not going to start now." Nancy, Anne, and I had a good laugh and Mama joined in. She always laughed with us even if she didn't know why we were laughing. After a good happy evening she would sleep well that night—an added bonus.

Remember that laughter is good for the body and for the soul as well.

Young Frankie and Clara Gentile,
whose mother Lynn was one of Mama's caregivers,
visiting with Mama Rose and playing with Duke I.

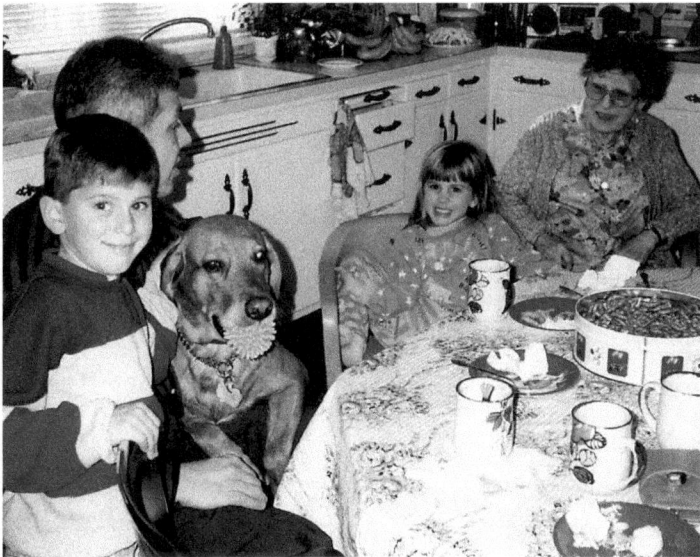

9

Seeing Major Changes in Mama

Another summer gone—another school year approaching—this was the rhythm of our lives. Mama had a good year with not too many visible changes. There were months when she seemed to be stable in her behavior, but then there were times when daily changes would occur and signal big losses in basic skills. I now began to see major changes in Mama. In spite of all the food she ate, she was losing weight due to her constant walking and the progression of the disease. She had depth perception problems too, and it was difficult for her to set a glass down on the table. If I handed her something, she often reached beyond and needed assistance. She found it difficult to use eating utensils. Almost every time, she would hold the fork or spoon upside down. When corrected, she still couldn't get the food onto the utensil. Mama found it easier to just eat with her hands. In spite of this she always tried to be neat and wiped her hands often, for she disliked being messy. Even when she was eating her much-loved spaghetti, she ate with her hands and made every effort to be as neat as she could. She also found it simpler to drink with a straw. Her tastes in food also changed. Even if she did not know what food she was eating, she still had definite ideas about what she liked or disliked. There were some foods she refused to eat, even though they were foods she had liked in the past.

In spite of her difficulty picking things up, Mama often took my knickknacks upstairs to her room throughout the day. Each night as she slept, I returned these items to the living room. One day on the QVC home shopping network, I saw a wax for sale that museums use to keep items in place. I ordered it and used it to attach everything permanently down to the coffee tables and cabinets. Mama got very frustrated trying to take these things upstairs and gradually forgot about this pastime of hers. This technique also worked to save my collectibles when the dog was flying through the room, tail wagging—nothing moved. When Laurie (Laurene Moran, our next caregiver) came to stay with Mama for the first time, she was amazed to find a coffee table that came furnished with knickknacks! We laughed about the items being waxed down and also about Mama's efforts to rearrange these items to no avail. Even the dog got a surprise when nothing fell over as he charged through the room.

Nighttime was often a difficult time for her (and me). If she wasn't sleeping, she was busy! When Mama was in a frustrated rage, she had strength and stamina beyond my comprehension for unending hours of night and day. In one of her screaming sessions, she would go up and down the stairs over and over, pacing back and forth, or spend time cleaning the house in great agitation. I was very worried that Mama's habit of going up and down the stairs would result in her losing her balance and falling because of her depth perception problem. Surprisingly, she never had a problem and could navigate the stairs with great coordination.

This was also about the time we learned that Mama needed diapers. At first this was so hard for her to accept, as well as for me. It came on her so suddenly. She would simply forget what to do. I remember thinking: I can't do this. "Well hello! There's no one else here." At all times I was careful to be aware of Mama's feelings. If she had an accident she would say, "I never did this before!" I would reassure her that all was well and then distract her and make her laugh. Distraction and laughter often worked to get us through embarrassing situations.

Duke was still Mama's special friend. He was always very patient with her, but his behavior seemed to indicate that he was becoming just a little weary. When eating, she shared food with her buddy. I recall many instances when he was covered with food and not liking it. If I gave Mama a dessert and the spoon was too large and I had to get another, I would return to find Duke covered with chocolate pudding. Often he would have cake crumbs on his head or juice on his coat. It was precious to see her share with him, but I don't think it was too comfortable for Duke. Once when I had parent conferences at school, my colleague Sister Anne Michelle LaMarre watched Mama for the evening. Sister was concerned because she knew Duke hadn't gone out, but she couldn't find him. When I came home, Sister was puzzled about where that dog was. I told her he was probably resting in the closet upstairs. He would open the closet door with his head and hide in the far corner. It was his way of saying, "I've had enough of Mama Rose." Even though Duke sat for hours at Mama's side and listened to her talk, with his back toward her sometimes, he did have a mind of his own, too, in dealing with Mama.

Sister Anne Michelle was one of my many friends who were wonderful with Mama and helped me out often. I really needed their assistance and was very grateful. They knew Mama's routine and always tried to make her as comfortable as possible. Once when my friend Sue was staying with Mama, they were both able to take an afternoon nap and all was quiet. But Mama woke Sue up to tell her exactly what time it was: It was time to eat. Sue laughed, got her some food, and also found Duke wrapped in an afghan and wearing a handkerchief on his head. Afterwards Mama said the Rosary with Sue, as she did frequently with me.

In the early days of Mama's illness, there had been occasions when I could bring her to school. I didn't bring her often, but when I did it was a pleasant experience. She used to love seeing the little ones. If they were playing, she was happy just to watch them. When I brought her to my classroom, they enjoyed talking to her and accepted the fact that she might not answer them. They wanted to read to her and they enjoyed her laughter. In March she had enjoyed coming to school for the St. Joseph Table where the children and their families would gather and share a meal. In June, she had also come to the kindergarten graduation. But now, she did not want to spend much time at school, and nothing could change her mind about staying with me in my classroom as I prepared it for the new school year. Gratefully, my many friends took turns staying with her so that I could get my room ready.

Our next caregiver was Lynn Gentile, a mom from school who had worked in a hospital. She was comfortable with Alzheimer's and willing to be with Mama for the school year. In the morning she brought her son Frank and her daughter Clara to my home. I drove them to school and Lynn stayed with Mama. After school, she brought Mama to school and I would take her home. Mama loved Lynn and her family, and the children were very loving with her. Lynn took Mama on many outings. Often she would take Mama to her own home and Mama played with Clara's dolls as if she were a new mother again, spending hours talking to the dolls. But then Mama would miss Duke and not be so cooperative. When she did consent to stay, she had a good time at Lynn's home because they also had a dog, but she wouldn't go every day.

> *The interaction between the elderly and children can be very positive for people with Alzheimer's at certain stages of their illness. Children are a wonderful delight for the elderly; they are lively and bring laughter and spirit and smiles for no reason. The children themselves benefit because if they are around the elderly early in life, they can learn to be very caring and understanding towards them. Within the family, it is very rewarding to have everyone involved in care. The more members of the family that are involved, the easier it is on everyone to care for your loved one. If the older children can relate to or watch your loved one for a while, it is a big help and usually a pleasant experience for all.*

Having seen Mama with Clara's doll, I decided to buy a doll for Mama to mother at home. She was content at first, thinking that she was babysitting. She was always very sweet holding the baby, mothering it, and talking constantly to it. She never saw the doll as her own child. She would reassure Duke that he was her first love: "I love Dukie, God loves Dukie." But she questioned what kind of mother would leave her child for hours, or why this mother never said a word of thanks. Mama kept repeating this so often that I saw this was a problem. How could I explain? So I decided that when Mama went upstairs, I'd put the doll in the closet and tell Mama the mother had come to pick up her baby. Unfortunately, this made her even angrier: "Not even a thank you." Mama wanted to tell this woman how she was neglecting her baby by leaving her at our house all day.

Soon it was summer again, a summer that seemed longer for me because I had to take each day as it came with the realization that Mama was failing more and more. I hoped to get through each day with a lot of faith and courage. I always knew her condition would get worse; but even though I expected her to have more setbacks as the years passed, I was sad when evidence of her failing skills actually became apparent. I wondered what direction life would take now. She was less aware of her surroundings and more confused about common items in the house, more in danger of getting hurt from simple items. She had more mood swings and outbursts of frustration. Perhaps this stage can be less stressful if there are many people in the home to help out with caregiving, but being an only child I found that this was all on my shoulders. Mama had asked me often where her other daughter was. I told her I didn't know, but if I found her I'd tell her it was her turn.

I missed the freedom to go on outings whenever I chose. Mama wanted to stay home more often, and her times with Duke were getting longer. If he came near my husband or me, Mama still got jealous and said constantly, "What, you don't love me anymore? God loves Duke and Duke loves me and God. Duke is a good boy." Many times she started prayers with "In the name of the Father, the Son, and the Duke!" Duke, however, was hiding more than before. At night, he wanted out of Mama's room; he would be scratching at the door: "Let me out!" She of course wanted him with her. Purely by accident, this situation resolved itself . . . to a point. I had bought a stuffed dog for a friend's daughter but found out she had one, so I kept it at home in a corner of the hall. He was all white and rather large. In a desperate moment, I gave the stuffed dog to Mama and told her it was Duke. She accepted the substitution and was happy talking to him all night. It seemed as if she didn't realize he was a stuffed animal. However, when I called Mama for breakfast the next morning, she in turn called the stuffed animal Duke to come. "Mama, this dog has to be carried downstairs." Her response was, "Then the h--- with him." This stuffed dog gave the real Duke a rest from Mama. She was happy to walk around with him and talk to him just as she did with the real Duke. There were also times when he was upside down. She fed the stuffed Duke many times a day. Once when my friend Kathy Bulger made some potato salad to share with us, Mama fed it to the real Duke but he was spitting it out. Kathy said to Mama, "I think he doesn't like potato salad." Mama responded, "He likes it. He ate it before," and proceeded to feed it to the stuffed toy. Stuffed Duke took many baths while Mama napped during the day or when she slept at night because he was often covered with food. Often on Friday nights, my friends Nancy Okerstrom, Pat Meyer, and Barb Stavnem came over to visit us. One time when they were sitting in the living room with Mama while I made coffee, I returned to find stuffed Duke covered in French onion dip. I teased them that there were three of them to watch Mama but Duke still got attacked!

Mama was losing interest in many of her favorite activities. She no longer read the newspaper. She still watched Channel 2 news because Mama thought that news anchor Linda MacLennan was so beautiful, but she really did not comprehend the news anymore. She even lost her interest in the Chicago Cubs. We used to watch the Cubs games on TV but did so less and less. She no longer understood what the score was or what it meant. We did have an opportunity to see a live game when my friends Pat and Nancy bought tickets to a White Sox game in the new Comiskey Park and invited us to come along. My first reaction was that we couldn't go to a Sox game because Mama was an ardent Cubs fan. But we finally decided to go because at this point Mama probably wouldn't recognize the teams who were playing . . . and she didn't. She was only interested in the snacks. When the Sox made a home run the fireworks went off and even that didn't get Mama's attention. We just kept the food coming. The young teenagers sitting in front of us did think we were a bit odd to say the least. They giggled as we tried to explain the game to Mama. Fortunately, it started to rain and we headed for home, because Mama would not have made it through nine innings.

Mama really did not want to go away from home. It used to be that if Mama was with other people or outdoors, she was happy. Now she only wanted to stay home. Every time we went out, Mama asked where we were going and why, and she showed some signs of fear and apprehension when we would prepare to leave the house. "Who lives here?" was the nice part of what she would say as we headed to the front door for an outing. If I answered that I did, she'd tell me that I never was any good even as a child! I assumed that she thought we should just stay home all the time because that's where we lived and we shouldn't leave – ever. Since this summer was extremely hot and had many ozone alert days, we did have to stay indoors more than usual. But we made every effort to have company around and to take her out so she could be entertained. Once we took Mama to the racetrack with my friends. The sun was bright, the park was beautiful, and the food was great, but she couldn't figure out why the horses were running away.

There were a few times when we did enjoy going out. On one summer afternoon we were invited to lunch by Kathy Stephens, a mother from school, and her daughter Brittany. Since I had not been to her home before, I needed directions. I was holding Mama's hand, my car keys, and the directions in hand as we headed out the door. Suddenly, Mama announced that she had to go to the bathroom. Every mom of a toddler knows how that goes, and I went back inside because Mama needed to be changed. Starting over, I put Mama in the car when I suddenly realized I didn't have the directions. Where could they be? Locking Mama in the car, I ran into the house to call my hostess for the directions again. Finally, ready to go, we were on our way, new directions in hand. The lunch was great, but Mama was edgy and wanted to head home sooner than I expected. I used every trick I knew to stall or distract her. Finally, I took her to the bathroom before heading home and to my surprise I found the original directions were in her diaper. I had to laugh and share the story with my hostess. On our way home, I needed to get something at the store for dinner. Mama was angry at the delay because she said we had been out too long already. She started swearing at me and made it very clear that Dukie needed her. I stood my ground: It was a quick trip through the store, but I finished my errand before heading home.

Mama was more cheerful on sunny days, as are most of us. On cloudy days, she looked for shoes, changed her clothes, hid food, and was very edgy. Nothing seemed to calm the waves. If we took a walk around the block, she seemed even more confused. She was also more restless and intolerant of her surroundings when evening came and the sun would go down. She would start to pace up and down the stairs, yelling, talking loudly, and showing increased confusion. The term doctors use for this behavior in people with Alzheimer's is "sundowning."

*Easter at the Hastings' home
with stuffed Easter Bunny*

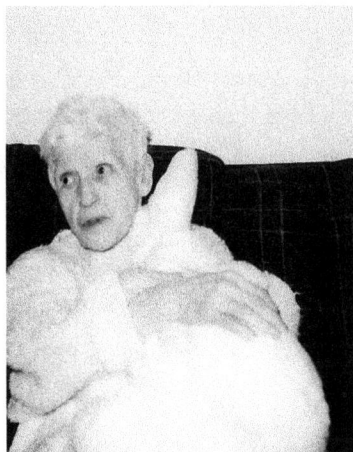

10

Still Enjoying the Holidays

Even though Mama's disease was progressing and there were many difficult times, we continued to live our lives as close to normal as we could, keeping her busy and including her in all activities. With each new day, there were many blessings. Holidays and celebrations made the time pass more quickly in a most pleasant way and Mama would get special attention, which she seemed to love. In preparation for any holiday, I always made every effort to decorate. Even if Mama didn't know what the decorations were for and I had to remind her about what event the holiday celebrated, I did think they lifted her spirits as well as ours. When I reminded her of stories about things we did in the past on those special days, she seemed to respond and be delighted to remember. Of course, she would also have brief moments of depression, for she would think back to when she was a child and would ask if her mom and dad would be around for the holiday. But she would soon recover and be happy again.

I remember one Halloween when my Bunco group decided to dress in costumes for our Bunco night at my friend Marie Scafa's home. I dressed Mama as Little Red Riding Hood and she looked precious. She seemed to enjoy wearing the outfit and being with company, and she played Bunco with the girls too. They were gracious to include Mama and once again, it was a memorable evening.

When Thanksgiving came around, I kept telling her that we were invited to my friend Lillian's home where there would be folks she wouldn't know or hadn't seen in a long time. I reminded her about how she used to love to cook the turkey dinner for this holiday in the past. All of this was in preparation for the day's outing. When the day came and we approached the house, she hesitated, but Rich was able to talk her through her anxiety. As soon as she arrived, she relaxed and was happy, and we were all able to enjoy a wonderful meal and several hours of talking and laughter. Our hostess, Lillian, was one of the St. Paul moms whose children I had taught. Lots of the families in the community were eager to help out once they learned of my situation.

Christmas was always a very special time, an occasion for many memorable moments. Weeks before, we would start to talk about this holiday and Mama seemed to enjoy seeing all the decorations. I was home with her all day during my Christmas vacation from school so I lit the tree during the day as well as in the evening. She seemed to respond to the old Christmas movies, especially *White Christmas*, and we sang a lot of Christmas carols that she remembered. Friends came over bearing Christmas gifts for Mama throughout the season. When she opened the gifts, she often didn't know what the gift was or its function, but the opening of the package made her smile and she always graciously said, "Thank you." Then she would offer the gift to Dukie.

One of Richard's favorite customs during the Christmas holidays was playing Santa for friends and community organizations. Mama was like a little child giggling with delight when she saw "Santa" heading out the door for one of his trips. He came every year to my kindergarten class, and one year she came for the class party too and enjoyed seeing my friend Jane sitting on Santa's lap. Another time I took her to the Elks Christmas Party to see "our" Santa, and she herself was willing to sit on Santa's knee like the other children. One year on Christmas morning, we went to Mass early and she was very prayerful and quiet. For our Christmas dinner we were invited to our friend Pat Meyer's home and Mama liked visiting with all the other guests. When it came time to sit down for dinner, however, she became edgy, and was eager to go home long before the meal was over. We tried many distractions, but nothing changed her mind about leaving. When we got home we noticed that she was not tired and definitely not at all ready to go to bed. She had just wanted to come home to be with Dukie and she was content again.

The coming of spring and Easter always brought new life to all of us. Once we were planning to celebrate Easter with the Hastings, a special family because their son Kevin, a kindergartner in my class at the time, invited us to share Easter with them. Mary Kay (Kevin's mom) knew Mama well and understood that it might be a very short visit. As it turned out, Mama had a wonderful time playing with the family's two big collies, Annie and Rosie. She liked the food and the atmosphere, but how she loved those dogs. Rich and I were really pleased that we were able to enjoy about four hours of good eating and conversation. The next year we celebrated with the same family again and they gave her a large white bunny to hold and talk to, so she was very content. There were little baskets of candy on the table that she liked, but she thought the Easter confetti decorating the tables was messy. She was very busy cleaning up the "mess."

Then there were parties: Confirmations, May crownings, First Communions, graduations. She was still able to enjoy all that celebrating. Her birthday fell on June 5th and was celebrated for many days and in several different settings and homes. This was wonderful. She would giggle and light up as everyone sang to her. One time I had a nice Italian dinner planned at Caesar's Restaurant. At the end of the meal, the waiters lit a candle on the cake and sang. "Mama, are you Italian?" "Yes, I'm Italian!" "Mama are you Catholic?" "No, I'm Bohemian." So we had a great belly laugh and a great birthday. Everyone laughing and singing always brought her delight.

At the end of each school year, the kindergarten children and I would put on a special graduation program for friends and families. Mama loved to come and see the children in their caps and gowns on the stage, reciting poems and singing beautifully. One year, Mama and I took a great picture at graduation with one of my kindergartners. As I put my arm around her I realized she wasn't wearing a bra! She had a lovely dress on and I didn't think anyone could notice except me. Like everything else, I can't explain how she got out of the house like that. How did she do all of these things? These were more moments to remember, some wonderful, some funny, others to ponder.

Mama Rose with stuffed Dukie

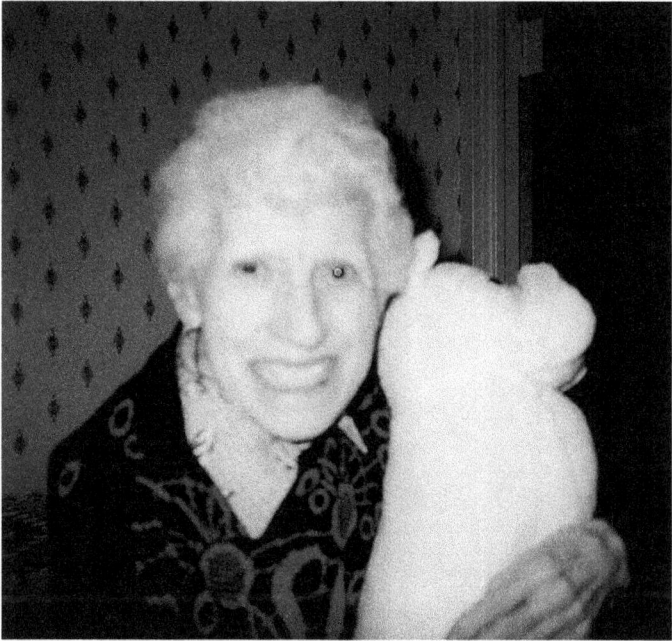

11

Coping with Mama's Physical Decline

The summer went by quickly and I saw that Mama's physical strength was failing more often. In past years, my caregivers would take her shopping and out to a park or for a walk. At home, they had prayed with her and watched television with her. Now that Mama was weaker, I was afraid that some of her outside adventures might not happen as frequently as before. As I started getting ready for the new school year, I had to prepare my classroom for the fall and find someone to stay with her. One day it would be my friend Barbara, another day it would be someone else. Mama was good with those who were watching her. If Mama didn't understand what they were saying to her, she always smiled. For whatever anyone did for her, she said "Thank you" to show appreciation. That made it easier to have folks help me out. Once my friend Mary Kay said that taking care of Mama at my home was like being on retreat since Mama Rose would often stay in her room and not come out. Not wanting to intrude, Mary Kay just let Mama do her thing; after all, Mama had her Duke to talk to. My friends not only took care of Mama but they helped me get my classroom ready, too. Nancy and Pat helped move furniture and Mary Kay gave all my bulletin boards a facelift. Actually, even though I was in charge, I had to leave Mary Kay and my other helpers alone in the classroom many times to return home and check on Mama.

Laurie Moran was going to be the caregiver for the new school year. She was a mom I came to know while I was teaching her three children. She was a wonderful person and I knew she would be terrific with Mama. She was very kind and thoughtful with Mama in so many ways. She laughed with her and kept her busy and happy. We worked out an arrangement where Laurie would bring her children to my home and I would take them to St. Paul of the Cross School with me for the 8:10 am start time. Her daughter Ellen, however, did not go to St. Paul's but to a District 64 school, and her classes started at 9: 00 a.m. To cover the 50-minute difference, Laurie would bring Ellen to our home and then take Mama with her to take Ellen to school. Ellen loved playing with Duke before school and in good weather would go out in the yard with him. This was not going over well with Mama, however, since Duke was her dog. And there were also times when it was time for Ellen to go to school and Mama would give Laurie a hard time, saying, "I'm not going." Laurie knew that with Mama and her moods, one often had to wait a short while and then approach the task again and hope that she would cooperate. Most times it worked.

Whenever my caregiver was ill or couldn't come, I had a backup person to care for Mama so I wouldn't have to miss school. Margaret Szajowski was one of my helpers who filled in and was wonderful with Mama too. Marge had a three-year-old at the time and I got a kick out of the fact that Mama thought the three-year-old talked too much. In reality, Mama wanted all the attention. If little Alexandra had a doll, Mama would take it away and we'd have a hard time getting it back. Marge took Mama out as much as possible. They were frequently out all day and very busy, going to places that were fun, like Chuck E. Cheese (Mama loved the pizza). When Mama came home from her day with the care person, she was ready for a good nap, but I would try to keep her awake in the evening so she would sleep that night. Luckily, I am a night person and could get all my chores done at night when everyone was asleep or at least in bed. This worked best if Mama was asleep, but many times she realized I was still up and about and she chose to join me. Then I just accepted the fact that some things wouldn't get done.

Mama needed more help with physical tasks and sometimes even had to be carried from one place to another. We were fortunate that Laurie was tall and strong. She lifted Mama whenever she needed to be moved during the day and Richard was there to help carry her at night. I especially appreciated Laurie's help in giving Mama a bath because I had been finding it difficult to get Mama into the bathtub. She was dead weight. Laurie was able to pick Mama up and place her on a seat in the bathtub and bathe her for me. This was wonderful because even though Mama often gave me a hard time about a bath, she was very cooperative with Laurie. At night there was the fun of getting Mama's teeth out and cleaned. When we finally got them out, we had the challenge of finding them in the morning to get them back in. Many a time Laurie started her day looking for Mama's teeth. We found them behind the dresser, under the mattress, in the closet. If we were not looking for her teeth, then we were hunting for her shoes!

Laurie was a lifesaver when Mama had a health crisis. Mama suffered from poor circulation and one rainy evening, when the pain was intense as she tried to walk, we decided to take her to the emergency room. Richard and my friend Mary Kay carried Mama to the car, which was parked on our front lawn so she wouldn't get too wet from the rain. The doctor gave her some medicine, but the next day the foot was more swollen and very hot to the touch. Laurie picked Mama up and took her to her usual doctor. He diagnosed poor circulation and told her to keep active, watch her diet, and avoid too much salt. Since Mama couldn't walk on that foot for some time, Laurie had to carry her to the table, to bed, and back to the couch. Luckily the swelling did not last too long and soon she was ambulatory, on the go, walking up and down the stairs as well as outside when the weather was good, but more slowly and not as angry as before. This made life a lot easier.

As Mama's physical strength declined, she became more loving and demonstrative. She was very affectionate and responded to hugs and handholding. This came so freely. She loved to be held and hugged and of course was loved by all of us. Laurie said that while there were many amusing moments with Mama, there were also times of peace and warmth. Sometimes Mama would nap during the day and rest her head on Laurie's shoulder. Then Duke had to join in right between them on the couch.

Despite her increasing weakness, Mama still had a lot of energy to continue walking a lot and keep going like the Energizer bunny. But her activities were often a source of concern to me, especially at night. Even though I knew she was very tired when she went to bed, I was never sure if she would sleep. I attempted to keep Mama so busy that she wouldn't have time for daytime naps and would sleep all night. During the day, I tried to have her string beads, keep walking till she was tired, fold towels and napkins over and over again, and dust furniture. But Mama had a way of responding when I least expected it if she didn't enjoy a task. She would give me a look and say, "Not doing this nonsense." We tried other ways of encouraging restful nights for Mama (and for all of us). Rich came home with a new mattress for Mama's bed, and Laurie gave Mama flannel sheets because Mama was always cold due to poor circulation. All these attempts did help a lot. However, Mama was often on nighttime adventures of her own, sometimes just talking nonstop to Duke but also roaming through the house, going up and down the stairs. I knew she couldn't get the doors open to the outside, but she could have fallen or hurt herself. I often felt blessed that her guardian angel was very busy watching over her because none of these terrible things happened to her. I put up gates to stop her from going down the stairs, but she managed to remove them. We put a lock on her bedroom door, but I never used it; I just couldn't lock her in for the night. I felt that she would be in terror if she wanted to go to the bathroom and couldn't open the door.

The doctor suggested an over-the-counter sleeping aid from the drugstore. At first this seemed to calm her wanderings, but not necessarily induce sleep. Then he suggested that he prescribe sleeping pills for her with the type and dosage determined by Mama's reaction to it. He cautioned us to monitor her closely because these medications could react with others she was taking. At first, even though she seemed fine, she was not sleepy, so he increased the dosage. But this didn't work either; one evening, she fell asleep on the stairs on her way to bed at a time when I was home alone with her and could hardly move her. It was very scary. Again he prescribed another medication, but this time she was uncoordinated. The medication seemed to linger in her body long after she took it and her days were crazy. I finally stopped following all his suggestions because her reactions were too erratic and dangerous. I took my chances and hoped that she'd start sleeping again on her own without a prescription.

Her wanderings were not limited to the night. On one sunny wintry day, I suggested an outing to Dominick's for some goodies. Even though Mama was content to stay indoors and doze in cold weather, she did enjoy an occasional trip outside and agreed to go shopping for some bananas with me. There was some snow on the ground but no ice; still, Mama refused to come into the store, deciding that she would wait in the car. I hesitated, but I knew I could lock her in securely and had done so on a few previous occasions. I rushed through the store and headed back to the car only to find it empty: Mama was roaming around, lost. I hurried to her side and she was very angry that "those so-and-sos" had left her in the car. I told her I didn't like the way THEY treated her either and she should come home with me. She agreed. Once again, I was blessed that she was not hurt or hit by a car or really out of my sight. I was also careful not to leave her alone again.

Mama Rose in earlier years
at Camille's wedding
with her youngest brother Jerry

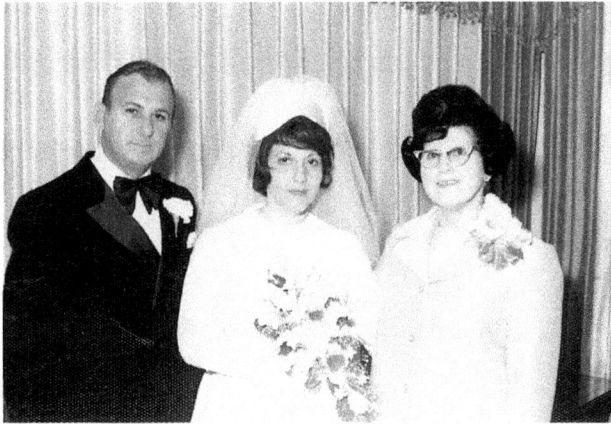

12

Meeting Mama's Relatives Again

Years after her diagnosis, the disease claimed another victim in Mama's family when we learned that her older brother Din also had Alzheimer's. Although the family had talked about his having symptoms similar to Mama's, it did come as a surprise to me when he was diagnosed. I took Mama to visit him a short time afterward. They didn't know each other, but I continued to have them visit each other. Mama had been close with this brother, too, and somehow the love that had once been between them still seemed to be present in some way. I was glad she didn't recognize his fate. He was as precious as Mama was, always praising God and having a great smile in the midst of his confusion.

Even though Mama did not recognize many people who had been a part of her life, she did remember her youngest brother Jerry who had lived with us for so many years. Mama took care of him almost all of his life, and she missed him terribly. She often was very angry about his not coming to see her and would frequently swear a blue streak at him. I could ease her mind by telling her that he was having a good time in Las Vegas. Remembering that he liked to try his luck, she would stop asking about him for a brief time. For his part, Uncle Jerry said that it was difficult to see her like this; he would cry and back out of coming for a visit. Although he and I were very close, we had many arguments over his not coming to visit her. When I would finally succeed in having him come, he would only stay for a short time and never want to be alone with Mama. He was that uncomfortable with her. It is true that everyone deals with this disease differently, but I found this to be the saddest part of the disease, that so many people are so uncomfortable with people with Alzheimer's that they ignore them, even though they love them very much.

I didn't hesitate in taking Mama to visit her brother who was suffering from Alzheimer's, but when her younger brother Jerry was very ill in the hospital, I refused to take her to see him. He was in a very serious condition and connected to many tubes. Anyone seeing someone like this can become very frightened and I didn't know what to expect in terms of Mama's reaction. I thought it would be better for her to remember him as he had been when she last saw him. Shortly after he went into the hospital, his heart gave way and he was gone from us forever. How could I tell her he died? What would be her reaction when she saw his body? How could she handle a funeral? I was anxious, and yet I knew we had to face this. I decided to act as if Mama were still her old self. When we went to the wake, she appeared to be unaware of the occasion. At the funeral parlor, she was looking for Uncle Jerry and couldn't comprehend that he was in the coffin: a blessing in disguise or sadness—I'm not sure. Mama had been having moments of reality and clarity about her brother and then those moments were gone. Both reactions were hard to bear and to watch her go through.

The anxiety of not knowing what to expect in any situation with a person with Alzheimer's is difficult because of the day-to-day mystery of the mind and its comprehension of reality. There is no clear pattern to determine when your loved one will be aware and alert and when all touch with real life will disappear.

Relatives at the funeral parlor who had not seen Mama in a long time said to me, "Oh, she'll remember me!" It was hard to make them understand that she knew none of us. They would try to have a conversation with her and were not convinced of her condition until they received no response or a wrong response. With concern and affection, I tried to explain Mama's condition to those who were once close to her and who didn't understand the disease. I tried to tell them some funny stories about Mama, so they could see she was still precious. I so wanted them to show love to her, but they only avoided her for the most part.

The funeral was long and difficult for me since I was very close to Uncle Jerry, who had lived with us so many years. He was like a dad to me, taking the place of my own father who had died when I was so young. Uncle Jerry made me laugh and we shared many special moments. He taught me how to drive and often lent me his car when I was in the convent. He would drive Mama out to see me from Berwyn every visiting day when I was at St. Xavier's College. He gave me away when I was married. He was my pal and my confidant.

At Uncle Jerry's funeral Mass, Mama entered St. Mary of Celle, the parish church she had attended for forty years and told me to make a wish—her custom whenever she entered a new church. Once again, I realized that Mama had forgotten so much of her past life and didn't even know her own church. However, she still remembered her precious custom of making a wish whenever she entered a new church. Often as I enter a new church, I laugh deeply and lovingly, remembering Mama's words, "Make a wish." She didn't realize this particular Mass was the funeral Mass for the brother she so diligently cared for and loved so deeply, but she still loved to go to Mass. She also had an awareness of the Eucharist, and after the consecration she turned to me and said, as she always did, "Going to Communion?" "Yes, Mama." That always seemed to make her smile and she said, "Me too," the usual response from Mama. For a long time even during her illness, she recognized the Eucharist as the Body and Blood of Jesus.

At the funeral luncheon, Mama ate very well and seemed content but very quiet. No one was really talking to her. Then all of a sudden she was ready to bolt home. Several days later when asking me about her brother, she finally comprehended that he had died, and she sobbed for almost twelve hours non-stop. Her understanding of his death did not stay with her permanently; time and again she would remember that he had died but then it would be gone from her mind. After some time had passed I continued to tell her that Jerry was in Las Vegas and she accepted that explanation and there were no more tears. As time went on she asked for him less often.

At one time, Jerry had asked Mama to help him invest in a land purchase in Arizona with two of his buddies. After his death, he left Mama his portion of the land. Because Mama had Alzheimer's, some of her siblings thought she should not have the land, so I retained a lawyer and fought to get her share of the property sale. In the end, with the legal fees that we alone paid for, Mama received nothing on the sale. Nevertheless, I was pleased that I had fought for Mama since she couldn't fight for herself anymore. She was still a person with dignity and had a right to the property. I would do it just that way again.

Mama Rose and TC

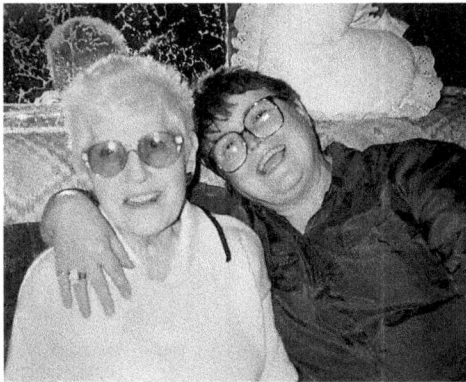

13

Looking for Daycare

As another school year came to a close, Laurie told me that she would return for the next school year but that she had been offered a computer job at St. Paul of the Cross School and would be working there three days a week. This was a great opportunity for Laurie, but it presented me with a dilemma: to find someone to take care of Mama on the days when Laurie couldn't be with her. I didn't want to lose Laurie for she was wonderful with Mama. Rather than hire another caregiver, I decided to start looking for a daycare for Mama for those days when she wouldn't be with Laurie. My friend Jane helped me with the search. We found a very nice place with a connection to a hospital and not too far from my school and home so that I could pick Mama up after school in a matter of minutes. The center had a variety of facilities. The general area had an alarm to prevent a patient from leaving the building, but they were able to roam about freely inside and choose their activities. The section for people with Alzheimer's was locked securely and well supervised. When Mama was evaluated, the process was a revelation to me, since I didn't realize how much Mama had forgotten, like her age, her birthday, the name of the day, the time. When she was totally lost on an answer, she just laughed. They decided that she would fit into the Alzheimer's group session.

The daycare session started at 9:00 AM and ended at 3:00 PM. I thought I should have Mama start the program before the end of the summer so that I could see how it would work out for her before I started teaching. It also gave me time to get my classroom ready for the new school year. As it turns out, daycare was not Mama's cup of tea. She gave me a hard time each day when she realized we were going to daycare. Then once we arrived, I had to slip away while they kept her distracted. When I picked her up in the afternoon, she couldn't get into the car fast enough and would tell me repeatedly that she wasn't going back there ever again. I knew she would receive good care at the center, but it was difficult to leave her when she was so against it. I would also need someone to take her to daycare once the school year started because I had to be at school much earlier than the center's start time. I still would be able to pick her up after school.

I was fortunate enough to find Betty, who cared for one of the students at St. Paul School. She would come to my home in the morning and spend some time with Mama before daycare and often take her out for breakfast. Betty was kind, had a great sense of humor, and enjoyed being with Mama. Knowing Betty from school, I trusted that this arrangement would work out just fine. I also knew that Mama behaved better with people other than me. As time went on, Betty saw many of the effects of Mama's Alzheimer's disease and the shift in Mama's moods. She often stayed at the daycare until Mama was settled down. Mama still didn't like daycare but she did like Betty. When she would see Betty arrive, she beamed as Betty got out of the car: "Here comes Mrs. Grafer!" It wasn't Margaret Grafer, my mother-in-law, but Betty reminded Mama of Margaret. Mama had always liked Margaret and they had been great company for each other.

Betty often spent the day with Mama if she was having a really bad day, when daycare would have been unbearable for her. Betty couldn't believe Mama's swearing on her bad days and was often saddened by her rages, but we did have some good moments and we shared some laughs over the stories Betty would tell me about her time with Mama. She said that when she would take Mama out for breakfast, Mama not only ate like a lumberjack truck driver but swore like one, too. Betty later told me it was a blessing for her to be with Mama because this experience helped her understand her own elderly parents even though they didn't have the disease. Mama was able to touch many people in many different wonderful ways. I knew that even on her worst days, she was a blessing for all of us.

Mama really did not like the daycare. The Alzheimer's unit was a very large room with a locked door and was staffed by more than one caregiver, but confinement was difficult for Mama since she liked to walk for most of the day. There were exercises, songs, music activities that Mama liked—but not there. Staff had planned activities for the people with Alzheimer's centering on socialization and the communication skills of the group. At this point, even on her best days, Mama wasn't one for social activities like Bingo at church or celebrations outside of the home. The activities at the center were focused on the ability of the most able patient and modified for those who were more severely disabled. It was a group activity, but Mama liked being independent. She would not participate at any level. They were only able to get a laugh out of her if they gave her individual attention. Much of the time there were too many patients and not enough workers to make individual attention for everyone possible. Now I was getting calls at school: "Come pick up your mother, she's causing trouble!" She was not a happy camper!

When most people think of people with Alzheimer's, they think of their walking off, getting lost, and not being able to find their own way back. In choosing a daycare, be sure that the facility is secure and has enough staff for the number of patients. Another thing to look for is a variety of activities that focus on the ability of the patients. These activities should give the person a sense of belonging and of purpose as well as an opportunity to communicate beneficially. If you are visiting and choosing a center, look at the people there. Are they happy? Do they participate in the routine and in the activities provided?

Sadly, Mama never liked the daycare, and the planned activities were of no interest at all to her. She didn't grasp the point of these activities, working with others or working for others, and she simply wouldn't enter into the projects. I had hoped she would find something there she could enjoy, but it never happened. The activities were planned in the form of games and Mama was not one for games. Clapping hands in rhythm, tossing a nerf ball or beanbags—these were of no interest to Mama. She would even walk through the circle when they were tossing the ball. She started each day wanting to go home. On a good day, the director would get Mama to dance and she'd like that activity and perhaps throw a ball, but mostly she sat by herself in a corner of the room. She was interested in a very old dog at the daycare, but he stayed in one room. Mama so wanted to play with that dog, but he didn't respond. She was used to her Duke. One day she said to me, "I think that dog is dead." She enjoyed a party when one was held for a special day but wouldn't make any decorations for the party. In her youth she had never been into crafts of any kind, and she was not about to start now. I saw the frustration the director was having trying to get Mama to participate. I had mentioned to him several times that first, she wasn't into games on her best day, and secondly, that she didn't understand the concept of the games. I asked them to let Mama do her own thing and she might come around slowly to participating, but this did not happen. The only time she was happy was when it was time to go home. Then she would beam and hustle to the car.

One afternoon, all the people with Alzheimer's and their caregivers took a field trip to a hospital. They had a sing-along and lunch when they arrived. As soon as I came to pick up Mama that afternoon, I was told that they had lost Mama in the hospital and she caused quite a stir. Mama wandered off and somehow got on an elevator that left her off near the doctors' area. So many doctors were trying to get a straight answer out of her as to where she belonged and who she was with! The daycare center director searched for her, riding the elevator and getting off at each floor in an attempt to find her. He finally found her on an upper floor talking to several doctors. He called down the hall saying, "She's mine, she belongs to me!" He laughed when I picked her up and said that at the time he was so relieved to have found her that he didn't realize how ridiculous he sounded. I really teased him several times afterwards about losing my

Mama. That's it—no more field trips for Mama Rose.

Once summer came again, I decided to stop taking Mama to daycare. On her last day, everyone celebrated her birthday. Betty made a wonderful cake for the folks at daycare and Mama enjoyed their singing and their good wishes. She was very happy. I remember thinking, could she possibly know this is her last day? The center staff was really sweet, telling Mama how much they would miss her, but in reality I'm sure they were relieved not to have to deal with her unhappiness.

The summer went by slowly, for there was not much Mama wanted to do. She was more agitated quite often, and even when she laughed she showed unrest. She became more stubborn and fearful at every outing we tried to enjoy, becoming very frustrated and often with unkind words on her lips. I took her to see her brother who was also suffering from Alzheimer's disease, but they didn't know each other much at this point. Sometimes a different face at home could make some difference. My friend TC would help me and keep Mama company while I slipped out for a break. Our nights were very disturbed, too. She was up at night walking the floors and often screaming in frustration. Almost every night was filled with anxiety. I knew I had to decide to place her in a nursing home before the new school year. Sleepless nights were no benefit to either of us. I prayed each day and night for guidance in making this very difficult decision, one I had hoped I would never have to make. I knew I would mourn the daily interaction I had with Mama, but I also knew that I had to realize my limits as well as free myself of guilt. Finally, I proudly came to realize all the responsibilities I had already taken on in Mama's care for eight years. I was grateful and amazed that I had kept laughter and love alive in her life.

*Sister Lois M. Rossi and Mama Rose
with Camille and Dukie*

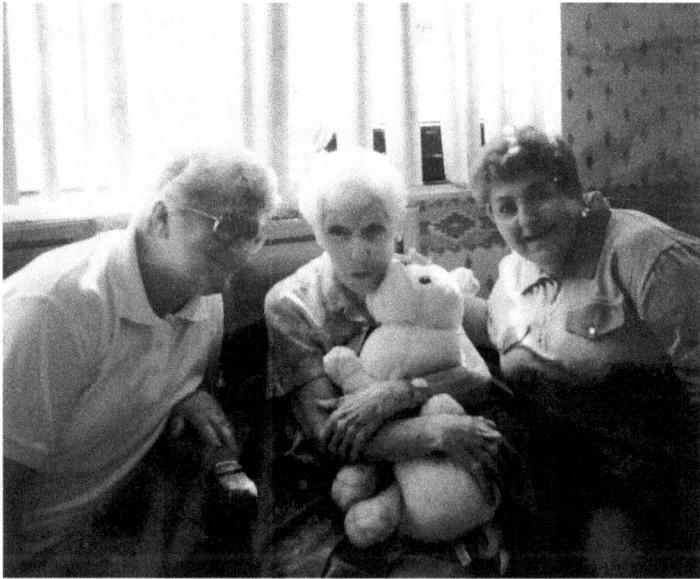

14

Choosing a Nursing Home

Once I had decided that the time had come for Mama to have twenty-four-hour care, my friend Jane helped me look into nursing homes. Fortunately, we could immediately get a feel for a place. If the place was lively, then it was usually outrageous in price and didn't accept residents who needed public financial aid (Medicare and most private health insurance programs don't pay for the custodial care of people with Alzheimer's). Many of the homes were very bright and decorated on the first floor, but the patients' floors told a different story: They hadn't been painted in a long time and the paint was a dull color. Curtains were drab and uninviting. We could sense gloom in the residents. Residents often did not appear to be clean and if there was a "smell" in a home, it meant that residents were not changed on a regular or as-needed basis. Activities were not going on anywhere. Laughter was not present in the halls, in the workers, or in the atmosphere. We looked to make sure the Alzheimer's floor was a locked facility, since residents have a tendency to roam or enter an elevator. To our dismay, the Alzheimer's rooms in some places were often bare and, worse, the residents appeared to be sedated to keep them quiet.

Let me share some advice from Sister Lois M. Rossi, a Franciscan Sister of Chicago and a nurse I referred to earlier who had a lot of experience with elderly patients. She was very helpful in giving me some guidelines as I went on my search for a good nursing home:

#1 Ask if the head nurses have been with the home for a long time. Are the staff members pleasant and do they love their work? If they have frequent staff changes, ask why.

#2 Check out the aides who are on the staff. Are they clean and alert to residents?

#3 Talk to residents if you can. You have to remember that most of them will tell you they hate the place because they don't want to be there, but you may be able to learn something. See if you can detect a sense of humor in the residents or other cues as to whether they are relaxed and feel safe.

#4 Look for nice bedding. We all know what that does to our spirit. Furnishings in halls and nurse stations should be bright and cheerful and clean. Bright colors lift one's spirits and show that someone cares.

#5 Look for a social director or an activity director who knows the residents by name. You will know by the residents' responses if being greeted is a common thing. Is there a schedule posted to indicate activities? Are the activities meaningful?

#6 Residents are always in the hall and watching the elevator. Are they talking? Are they friendly? Are they clean and dressed for the day? Are they alert? Or do they seem to be drugged?

#7 Meals are always difficult to judge, for you might visit on an off day when they have liver (although if you like liver, that will change your impression of the place). At mealtime you want to see if residents are assisted in their eating, if the surroundings are clean, and if the food is appetizing. On the Alzheimer's floor, there should be finger food available so residents can be independent if they have difficulty with utensils.

#8 Ask about special days or celebrations and if the residents have special treats. If they do have treats, ask when and how often. Be alert to the surroundings. Are the halls decorated for whatever holiday is approaching? Are meals reflective of the holiday and posted for visitors to see? Talk to other visitors. All of this is an indicator that in this home, someone cares.

#9 Does the home offer an opportunity for residents to express their faith whatever it may be? Do they allow religious wall hangings or other religious items in the rooms? Do people seem to have their personal touches in the rooms?

I was impressed with a nursing home that was close to my own home in the northwest area. There was no foul odor in the halls, no foul smells throughout the place. The staff was friendly and eager to help in any way they could. While I was concerned that many of the aides only spoke Polish, I learned that they knew the English they needed to care for and relate to their patients. I also learned that the aides' job did not really involve extended conversations with the patients because they never had much time to converse with the residents. I was also pleased that this home was bright and truly very clean. It had a very cheerful and friendly atmosphere and was also very conveniently located for me so that I could visit often throughout the day and at odd times. After visiting a number of homes and after much consideration and prayer, I made my choice.

The director was very helpful to me and gave me peace of mind with her guidance, and the staff was sensitive to the fact that this was the most difficult decision I ever had to make. The head nurse had been there for almost 20 years, one of the guidelines I thought to be very important. She greeted all the residents by name and they seemed happy to see her as she appeared on the floor. She was personable and made me comfortable when I was talking to her about my concerns.

I still went through mental anguish, asking myself many questions when I was alone. Am I being selfish by placing Mama in a nursing home? Is this my last recourse? Would Mama understand this move? How could I get through this terrible time of leaving her in someone else's care? I was fortunate to have strong support from my husband and close friends who encouraged me and assured me I was making the right decision. By this time, Mama was roaming about all night long and I wasn't getting enough sleep to be effective at work. Teaching has always been a passion with me and I felt fortunate that I could be a teacher. I knew I couldn't afford to neglect my teaching responsibilities in the classroom or discontinue working. I knew it was time for Mama to move to a nursing home, but I still hesitated in making the immediate and obvious decision. Memories of daycare kept coming back to me over and over. She had so hated daycare even though the staff there was very kind; it just had not suited her personality. Going there was so painful for Mama, and I was afraid that this move now to a nursing home was going to be terrible for Mama, too. I had no reason to think otherwise since now Mama showed more irritation to most things I had planned for her daily routine. Somehow, with lots of faith, I prayed and finally reached my decision.

Mama Rose
with Camille and Dukie

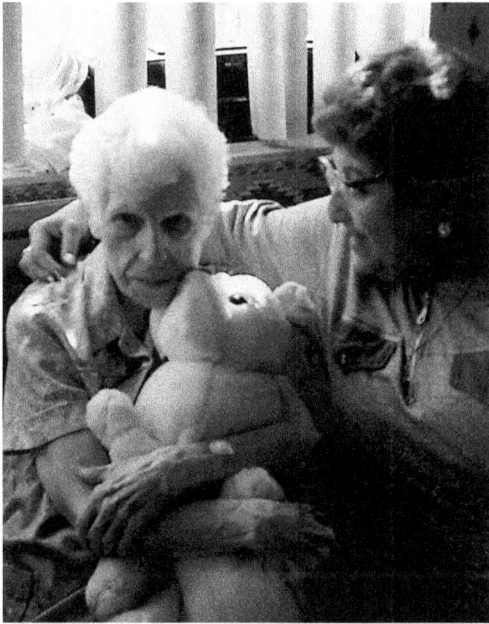

15

Moving Mama to the Home

*The names of all residents, as well as details
about location, have been changed to protect
the privacy of Mama's companions in the home.*

In June of 1996, I decided to move Mama to the nursing home. The home had a locked facility for the residents with Alzheimer's, and they were willing to take a person who was on public aid supplemented by the resident's social security check and any other assets. I felt blessed that all was moving along in such a positive way, and that this place had lots of advantages for me and Mama. I started the paperwork with confidence that this was the only choice I had at this time. The home director helped me fill out all the forms and, since Mama already was on public assistance, guided me through the process. They also were willing to take Mama into the home before all the forms were processed by the state. I wanted to get her settled before school started again, and the summer would offer me an opportunity to visit during the day and for longer periods of time. It would also give me more opportunities to get her outdoors during the day and to really get to know the true spirit of the home.

The day finally arrived when we would have to leave for the nursing home. I felt lucky that Mama would be taking her "stuffed Dukie" to hold, love, and talk to. I was grateful that Richard came with us and took Mama to the car. I really appreciated that Jane offered to be with us too; she had been so supportive and helpful in finding this place. I needed all their support and encouragement to make this move less traumatic for both Mama and me. I worried and prayed so often over this move—so I don't know why I was so surprised when Mama was terrific in settling right in. If Mama was consciously aware of her new surroundings, I didn't know. She immediately took stuffed Dukie in hand and started walking back and forth down the home's long halls. After I set up her room, hanging up her clothes, placing a new plant next to her bed and a statue of the Infant of Prague on her dresser, I said, "I'll see you tomorrow, Mama!" I gave her several hugs and kisses. "Okay!" was all she said and down the hall she went, talking to Dukie. I realized that because she loved to walk, she was content to start on her new journey by walking down every hall. I had been setting up a variety of activities for her but she only wanted to do some simple walking. Richard, Jane, and I decided it would be best to leave at that moment on a happy note. As we were leaving, a woman named Jenny told us she was in charge of the floor. I proceeded to tell her about Mama and then realized she was wearing a wristband. She was one of the residents! We left to the sound of laughter.

The head nurse had told me to feel free to call later to see how Mama was doing after we left her. I needed to know she was adjusting to her new surroundings. I called, and to my surprise they told me she was doing fine. She gave no one any trouble and was now in bed starting to fall asleep. They reassured me that they would keep a close eye on her all night. I talked with the head nurse several times that night. I prayed in thanksgiving that all seemed to be going very well.

Before lunch the next day, my friend Mary Kay and I went to visit Mama. She was very busy walking up and down those wonderful long halls with her Dukie, but we did manage to get her to sit and enjoy her lunch. This is when we met Marie, who had been a beauty queen years ago. The nurse told us that Marie had won a beauty contest in the late 1920s and that everyone on staff referred to her by her title, "Miss Hometown." She was a feisty lady and made us laugh with her tales about the "food" and "this place." After lunch, Mama and Dukie left the table and were back to their walking. So we started to sing with the residents who were still sitting at the table. It was then we came to know that it was Lorraine's birthday because there was a balloon tied to her chair to celebrate her special day. Mary Kay and I started to sing and when Lorraine joined in, we realized immediately that she could sing beautifully. We were able to encourage her to sing several other songs, among them the "Ave Maria" in Latin. We were moved to tears hearing her sing to our Blessed Mother so beautifully in prayer. We came to know that she had made some recordings in her earlier years. We had a wonderful visit for a few hours with several of the residents as well as with Mama. We had to hustle to keep up with her as she walked up and down the halls, smiling and talking away to Dukie, so we left with a wonderful feeling of peace. I knew then that I had made the right decision, for Mama was very content and, while glad to see me, was not at all upset to see me leave. I hoped that this would now be her daily view on life. I went back that evening to see her and she was still walk-

161

ing but did sit down and visit with me. She was tired and they were ready to get her into bed. When I called later that night they told me she was sleeping soundly.

Life at home was quieter after Mama left our home because our Duke was never quite the same. He remembered her and would not go into her bedroom or jump up on the couch where he had sat with her everyday. We knew Duke was a terrific dog and we sympathized with his loneliness, so soon after Mama left, we brought in another dog to keep Duke company while we were at work, a golden Labrador, gentle and sweet. Duke tolerated the other dog for a long time but then decided to accept him and they eventually became friends. When we brought Mama to our home for a visit, she would say, "Oh, there are two Dukies. Wow!"

Halloween at the nursing home

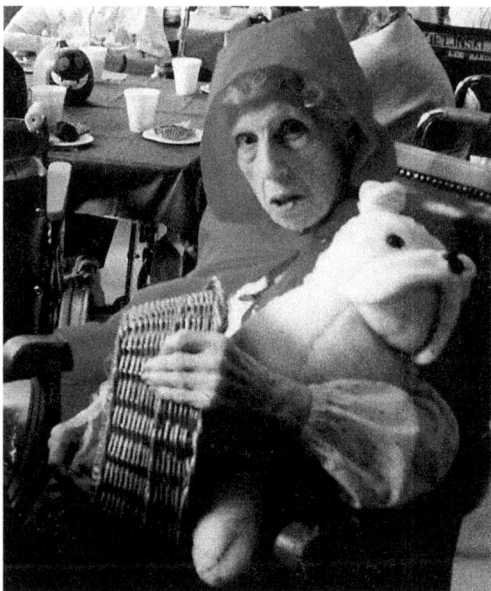

16

Visiting Mama & the Other Residents

Mama's first day at the home was the beginning of her new life and, for me, the beginning of many pleasant visits to her and her fellow residents. I went during the morning and sometimes returned in the afternoon. I went in the evening around dinnertime to make sure she was eating. They never knew when I would appear and I was able to stay for a long period of time. I became familiar with the routine and was very pleased with the care the residents received. Workers visited the patients in the morning and did activities with them. Some patients were also able to participate in activities that were set up on another floor for all the residents. Those in wheelchairs would be helped by the nurses onto the elevator for some events, and those who were ambulatory could go downstairs more often. Of course, many residents were too disruptive to be taken downstairs and some were in beds on a regular basis.

The Alzheimer's floor residents had a midday treat of chocolate milk, Ensure (a vitamin-enriched drink like milk), and crackers; in the evening, they had a snack of juice and cookies. Bingo and ice cream socials were made available every day. Mass was available on Friday afternoons. The home was always beautifully decorated for every holiday, and there were special parties at various times of the year. One summer event was a grand setup in the parking lot, a Hawaiian Party with dancers. There was also Bingo Night, a Song Fest, and many special events for the residents to share with their families.

It is best to visit at different times. You can then really get a feel for the home and the staff's behavior with the residents at all times.

I came to know the staff very well on all the shifts. I made sure that I expressed my appreciation for all their service and kindnesses to Mama and I found that any complaint I had was rectified quickly. My requests were simple: I wanted my Mama clean and comfortable, and I also made it very clear that she had to have Dukie with her at all times. The nurses and aides seemed to love Mama and did look out for her. They would relate a funny story about Mama or laugh as they told me about her talking to Dukie and swearing at everyone while walking down the halls at full speed. Sometimes when I came in they would warn me she was having a bad day. I'm also sure she gave them a harder time than they let on to me.

The staff made sure that communication between staff and each resident's family was ongoing by holding conferences to discuss how the resident was doing and to answer any questions the family might have. Most of the staff found Mama to be very pleasant and easy to work with every day. When she had an "angry" day once in awhile, they did not disturb her but let her rest. I used to have difficulty getting her out of her bad moods and the workers also found this to be true. Then the next day she would be her pleasant self and our visits were happy. I always made sure to compliment the unit's workers and nurses to the main office for their care of Mama.

It was no surprise to hear from staff that Mama had difficulty participating in the day's activities. When I had a school day off, I went to see the activities they planned, and they were much like the ones at daycare. My presence didn't help Mama respond any better. She was "very busy" walking and talking to Duke. She would sit in the circle but not participate. The activity director on the Alzheimer's floor was wonderful with Mama and always made Mama giggle with laughter. She would comb her hair, polish her nails, and put makeup on her. She even visited Mama on her time off. I was so appreciative for the care she gave Mama.

When I went to the home at mealtime, I observed how well the residents were fed and cared for every day. I was happy that the meals were very healthy and appetizing because food in most institutions can be very dull and unappealing. Many of the residents who couldn't have salt or sugar were accommodated with the special diets they needed; others who had difficulty chewing were served soft food. Many of the residents also needed to be fed because they couldn't feed themselves. All were taken care of very thoughtfully by the staff. When I visited, I also noticed what was apparently a mealtime custom: Many residents who were in wheelchairs would take their "favorite spot" at the table at least thirty minutes before the meal was served. I learned that I had better not sit in that spot for a meal or a visit because they would become upset. Mama needed to eat well because she was walking almost nonstop. In addition to the regular meals at the home, I made sure Mama also had some special treats. She loved her Italian goodies which were perhaps a little heavy on the olive oil, but she was so fond of them that my friend Maria Pohlson made several plates of Italian pasta for Mama and added meatballs. I would put these plates in the freezer and several days a week I would warm a plate and watch Mama enjoy her favorite food. Maria was so pleased with Mama's look of joy when she saw the mostaccioli being served. This she ate very well, but at other times it seemed that Mama only sampled her food. I also brought cannoli and milk shakes so that she would have other special treats because she always enjoyed her sweets. Mama fed Dukie everything she ate, especially the vegetables which she didn't like. Poor Dukie! One day he was on a chair with a bowl of beets in front of him and of course he was all red. "Mama, how come Dukie has your beets?" I asked. "That's what he wanted!" was her response. Duke was so red from the beets that I was concerned because he really needed to be cleaned. I was lucky to find another stuffed Dukie exactly like the original. Now I could switch Dukie and take the dirty one home to wash. When I returned with Dukie all clean and white, the head nurse asked me how I got all the red out. I told her I threw Dukie in the washer and dryer. One of the residents was listening and scolded me for being so cruel to that wonderful dog. I immediately responded that I put him in the tub for a bath. Well, she was happy to hear that. We laughed and I was forgiven. After that, every three or four days Dukie got a bath. Somehow Dukie lost an ear and to this day I don't know how it happened. Mama didn't love him any less.

From my reading and research, I learned that in general, nursing homes are frequently short-handed and the pay scale for aides in particular may not be the best. There is often a frequent change of aides who have the very difficult job of performing the undesirable tasks of bathing, changing diapers, shaving, and dressing the residents. Sometimes aides may have limited English and little opportunity to advance. Knowing all this, I was grateful that many of the staff on the Alzheimer's floor had worked there for a long period of time. So many of the aides were exemplary persons who worked very hard and were eager to help Mama in any way. I observed that those who were constantly working on the Alzheimer's floor were folks that were very pleasant and had a sense of humor. Anyone who might be impatient would never make it on this floor. I often praised the staff for their work, knowing how difficult their work had to be day after day.

I went to see Mama daily, sometimes twice a day and at different times, to be sure she was fed and clean – and she was. Mama always welcomed me with a big smile. I could get her to settle down with something to eat most of the time. When I wanted to be just with Mama, we would go to the far end of the hall for a visit. As we sat at the end of the hall one day, men were on the outside cleaning the windows. Mama thought they were her brothers and went to the windows to tell the workers off: "Where the h--- have you been you s-- of a b----!" Needless to say, they were shocked, their mouths hanging open, but I enjoyed the humor of the situation.

The "girls" and "fellows" on the floor soon became my family to visit as well as Mama. If someone did not feel like being sociable, there were always so many more who were glad for a visitor. I was always greeted with a big smile by Mama as well as by the other residents when I appeared on the floor. They came to recognize me as soon as I got off the elevator. The residents were mostly content to sit for hours in the halls and stare at walls even though they had their morning activities, three meals, and snacks. So I loved to spend time with them and get them singing and talking to help them pass the time. My friend Maria remembers how we would bring a tape recorder and the residents would all sing along to simple songs like "Row, Row, Row Your Boat." They were always so warm to me and wanted so much of my attention that I often had to remind them that I had come to see my Mama who was walking the halls with her Dukie. "Oh, is your mom here?" they often asked in surprise. I frequently brought treats for Mama and the other residents (staff approved of course)—a box of cookies, perhaps, and by offering them to the residents, I came to know their names. In time, I came to know their different personalities as well. I also came to know those who had difficulty at different times. Some were angry in the evening but not in the morning. Some were consistent day and night. Some were enraged at bath time. Some were happy most of the time.

Unfortunately, there were other visitors to the home who told me they found it scary to visit, especially when they would see a resident talking loudly or screaming in someone's face. They were afraid of the residents and refused to come back for another visit. As time went on, I became aware that this feeling was apparently not unusual, for most of the residents didn't get visitors at all. Some of the relatives openly admitted they had difficulty visiting their loved one. Some just had excuses that they expressed to the staff; they would call and ask that the resident be told they couldn't come on that particular Sunday. When I inquired further, a staff member told me many of the residents went years without any family member visiting them. If a decision had to be made for a resident's care, the staff had to call the family for approval because they never saw them. It gave me great sadness to see the absence of visitors. No matter how the residents were in the past, the disease had now made them different people. It is true that some residents were difficult to deal with. On a few occasions I did see a resident screaming at the visitors, not wanting to see them, and the family left in great pain. Sometimes a resident was screaming at anyone in sight to leave them alone, even though after a while they would be happy to see a friendly face once again. I thought it unfair to make a judgment about a family member's lack of response or responsibility for the resident because much was unknown to me. But I wanted to do as much as I could to help the residents have a more pleasant life. I saw a possibility for service, to help the staff by making more hands available to help the residents on the floor—more people to reach out to many of these folks. So I decided to bring my family of friends with me to visit Mama and the other residents.

> As you go into a nursing home, you may see the residents with Alzheimer's sitting in the hall. They are staring out at you and no one is communicating. They seldom have much to say to each other. Yes, this is sad. What can you do? Start to talk to them and you will discover so many different personalities. You find that their preciousness is not lost. They still have something to share with you, even if it is just a smile or a laugh. On the other hand, a person with Alzheimer's might also become very uninhibited and sharp enough to be disturbing to some people. They may also try to escape from the illness when they resort to sleeping a great deal. Remember to try to help them anyway.

My many friends came to visit the residents with me when they could. When I would bring them, they were so impressed with the home, especially with the residents. All those in the Alzheimer's unit became our family. We would entertain the entire floor and since we had a regular circle of visitors, we had many moments of shared laughter. We were immediately rewarded by the residents' gracious response. Our visits became quite elaborate and fun. We knew the residents by name and enjoyed each individual personality. We tried to be creative in making our visits special for the "gang" on the Alzheimer's floor. We took them downstairs to the yard and pushed their wheelchairs around the grounds. We took them to visit the ice cream parlor. We sang with them. We always had cookies (staff approved) to pass out, and that opened the door for each resident to be talkative. Several of us would bring ice cream bars or all the makings for a Fudge Sundae or Dunkin' Donuts Day (all staff approved and in keeping with dietary restrictions). We even planned a tea party for one of the Irish residents for her 93rd birthday; we fixed a lovely decorated table downstairs with good china and flowers and served Irish soda bread. We played Bingo with vanilla wafers or marshmallows for markers (since the residents ate the markers). We even planned a garage sale during which the residents could pick an item they wanted. We made sure we had items for the men, too. I had so many spiritually rewarding moments that I was sure we were on a most important mission. The Lord said, "Whatever you do to the least of My brethren, you do to Me." I knew that Mama was here for a good reason. Being able to connect to these folks and bring smiles to their faces made wonderful memories with the "guys and girls."

We also started to say the Rosary with the residents. Many of them knew the prayers by heart. I passed out glow-in-the-dark rosaries and most wanted to wear them. Even though some of our circle of residents saying the Rosary were not Catholic, they still wanted to participate. Seeing them engaging in a group activity like this made me thankful that my friends and I had been able to help them. When we prayed the Rosary, Mama sometimes prayed with us, but at other times she'd walk off saying, "Did that all my life." She would make a point of walking through our circle as we prayed in order to be noticed. After the Rosary, we had a singing fest and I could get Mama up to dance. It was another precious time with her and she showed her pleasure with her usual giggle. It was certainly God's work.

The residents enjoyed our visits so much that I thought it would be a good idea to include children. I took my class list of kindergartners and arranged it so that over the course of several holidays, each child would be able to pay a visit to the home. Most families were encouraging in letting their child come to visit. I made it clear to parents that this was the Alzheimer's floor and could be frightening at times with residents sometimes screaming non-stop. I explained that the reason I was taking the children to this floor was that of all the folks in the home, these residents had the least number of visitors. They also were the most childlike and would fuss over the little ones. There were a few families through the years who wouldn't allow their child to come, but most were happy to give their child this opportunity. Some of the kindergartners would be very quiet and shy but most were very outgoing. The parents came too, so we had a nice big group of people to visit with the fifty or so residents on the Alzheimer's floor.

I planned my first visit with the children for Halloween, which was the easiest because the children were in costumes and weren't afraid. I called ahead of time so the staff would have the residents gathered in the family room. We put on a little program and then passed out treats and talked with the folks. It was a fun and successful visit. The residents made a big fuss over the children, and the children and their parents were enthusiastic about visiting these folks. One little boy, Kevin, said, "Hello Mama Rose!" when he recognized my mother. She was in her walking mode, so she replied "Can't talk to you now, little boy, I'm very busy." Kevin and I laughed and so did Mama. The home also had a Halloween party so Mama wore her Little Red Riding Hood outfit at both parties. All the staff raved at how cute Mama was in her outfit and about Dukie who was the Big Bad Wolf.

I was very pleased with the positive reaction on the part of the residents and the children, so after that first visit, I planned many others that were equally successful. When I would bring the kindergartners, the residents were always so happy to see the little ones in their special outfits and to hear their songs. We brought treats and conversation and brightness to the day and, of course, Mama had to tell the little ones about her Dukie.

Knowing that the residents enjoyed having the children in for a visit, I spoke to St. Paul's eighth grade teachers. They encouraged the eight graders to come to the nursing home because the students had to perform community service for a certain number of hours in order to prepare for their Confirmation. The older children were a little more unsure of the task but were surprised at how well received they were by almost everyone. John, one of the residents, was in his mood of wanting to be alone and chasing everyone away until he saw the children talking to the other residents. Then he saw how much fun they could be and wanted to be included. The eighth graders really liked the experience and talked about these folks to their family and the other students at school, encouraging other students to come see what the home was like. And so the students began to visit on several occasions. The youngsters came up with their own ideas of things they could do or bring to make the residents happy. One of the eighth graders brought her dog, who was a big hit, for the residents loved animals and this was a dog they could hold, too. Another time one of the eighth graders made turkey ornaments for each resident, and one student brought old jewelry for the ladies to wear and keep. Most of the youngsters came because it was a kind thing to do regardless of the fact that they had service hours to earn. It was a value their parents believed in and a good service to give to others. Soon others were visiting the residents because of the stories they heard from the St. Paul students. My friend Mary Kay started to bring her family of boys. She wrapped presents for the folks at Christmas time and even dressed up as the Easter Bunny in spring. My friend Michele Whalen also came to visit with her family.

Mama was consistently funny and precious. She was much loved and she responded to that love with warm hugs and kisses. The staff responded to Mama, too, for most of the time she was pleasant and quite funny. She wasn't a quiet and shy person any longer. She had a new routine that included fake crying. I'd ask her who she was and she wouldn't remember her name and say, "I don't know." I would then say, "Okay, then if you don't know your name, I'll call you Madame X." She'd do the fake cry, "No, don't call me Madame X!" We roared when she'd do this. I'd tease her and she'd repeat that fake cry. She couldn't remember exactly who I was either. If I told her I was her daughter, she'd look at me in a strange way and tell me I was too old to be her daughter. Her memories of her daughter had to be of me as a child. She did know me as a good person and a friend, for she always smiled beautifully whenever she saw me come out of the elevator. That was enough for me. Titles are not that important. At the end of each day, always on Mama's lips, was "Dukie is a good boy, I love Dukie and God loves Dukie." Then we'd sing "You Are my Sunshine" to Dukie and after she laughed, she'd cry her fake cry and say "No more."

Dukie was a big hit on the Alzheimer's floor. The residents thought Dukie was the best dog. He didn't bark and never left a mess on the floor. Dukie was so well cared for by everyone as well as by Mama. Knowing how loved Dukie was, I asked the kindergarten class to donate any stuffed animals they no longer wanted as a nice gift for the patients on Mama's floor. When all the donations were collected and I took them to the home, the residents were delighted to pick one out and hug it. Even the aides asked for a stuffed animal. Much to my surprise, the next day I didn't see some of the stuffed animals. I discovered that the residents of the Alzheimer's floor often hid things they treasured because others sometimes took things they mistakenly thought belonged to them. There were times when I came to visit Mama and her Dukie was missing. Then I would look into the residents' rooms until I found him. One resident would take him away from Mama and hide him. Whenever I found her with a Dukie in her arms and made it clear to her this was my Mama's dog, she would tell me, "I'm the one that gave her that dog." We laughed. Yes, but that is Mama's Dukie now.

A problem can arise in all nursing homes because the residents may see something they thought was theirs and take it, not really aware of what they are doing.

The residents themselves are often misplacing some-thing and forgetting where they had left it. One way to solve this is to mark the resident's name on the object with a marking pen in large letters. The staff is always sympathetic, of course, and ready to help, but fami-ly members and friends are often the best resource to identify the missing objects.

Mama often didn't notice when something of hers went missing (unless it was Dukie) and I did mark her belongings so that they would stay around a little lon-ger, but eventually something might still disappear and I'd go hunting for it. At my own home, there was a lim-ited amount of space where something could be lost or misplaced, but at the nursing home, there were so many more places where something could be lost. Sometimes Mama's clothes would not be in her closet but I would see them worn by another resident! I was most upset when Mama's teeth were misplaced. The first few times I was lucky to find them in her drawer or in a glass in the bathroom. About a year and a half after she moved to the home, her top denture was missing and she was hav-ing difficulty eating. I tried to get a dentist to make her a new set but encountered many obstacles. First, Mama would be frightened when getting a mouth impression. Secondly, she wouldn't be able to tell us how they fit or if she had any pain. Finally, Public Aid didn't look fa-vorably on paying for new dentures because it was costly and often the patient refused to wear them. Even when I was willing to pay for a new set, the staff made it clear that from their experience they thought it would not be a good investment.

Her glasses would often be missing too and then I would be on the search. Like the teeth, they'd be lost and found many times. They might be in a drawer, in a shoe, or on another resident. The staff assured me they would hide her glasses at night and put them on her in the morning. It was difficult to know if the glasses were comfortable on Mama; why was she taking them off after she was dressed? I finally decided to take Mama for an eye exam. The doctor tested her for any diseases of the eye but couldn't change the prescription because Mama was unable to read the letters or tell him if what she saw on the chart was blurry or clear. So we only had the one pair of glasses and were not sure they were suitable.

Mama's days at the home were pleasant, but occasionally we would take Mama on an outing. Once, my friend TC and I decided to take her for a ride. While I was busy talking to some of the residents, TC took Mama to the car and opened the back door on the driver's side to let Mama in. To our surprise, Mama couldn't figure out how to get in the car. Mama only knew how to get in on the passenger side! I was laughing so hard, I made no effort to help TC who was laughing too but also frustrated and asking me to help. Another time when Richard and I took her out for a visit, she couldn't remember how to go up the stairs and Richard had to carry her into the house. Even though she seemed to enjoy our outings, the visits outside of the nursing home were getting fewer and fewer because they were more difficult for Mama. I concluded that if a skill was not used regularly, it soon was lost.

Mama Rose at the nursing home

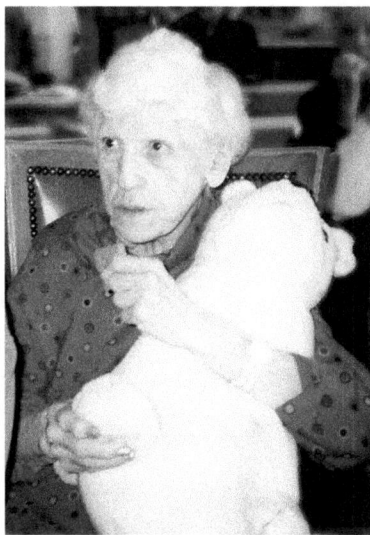

17

Learning the Residents' Stories

I have so many wonderful memories of our time with the residents at the nursing home. They were all very special persons. Those on the Alzheimer's floor were in some cases only shadows of who they had been before, both in actions and in their speech. The staff always tried to make sure that the residents' behavior was not upsetting or offensive to anyone, but occasionally my friends and I would be in for some surprises.

> *It is important whenever visiting people with Alzheimer's that you are always calm and nonjudgmental and that you remember to treat each person with respect, recognizing the dignity each one has as a fellow human being, and remembering that it is the disease that has robbed them of their control and sense of propriety.*

Upon entering the home, I would invariably run into Arlette, a first floor resident, who was walking down the halls with her walker. Her walker had a basket which usually held a carton of milk and dishes filled with food

185

from her meals. Arlette was on her way outside in all kinds of weather to feed the cats who came around the parking lot. She loved animals and was always busy looking out for them.

Beatrice was one of the smokers I'd see outside who I loved to tease. She was a sweet lady and very sharp. She was also Italian, and while she loved Italian food, she also loved Fannie Mae chocolates. She had worked at their factory for many years when she was younger and just a few chocolates could make her very happy. She lived on the first floor, for though she was self-sufficient, she was in a wheelchair. She hated being in the home and never had a good word about the place. She'd actually make me laugh because she was so critical about everything. No matter what day it was, she would say she was not feeling well but was full of the dickens and it was really easy for me to make her laugh.

Of course, most of my memories are of the residents on the Alzheimer's floor. As I said earlier, one of our special persons was Marie, whom everyone called by her beauty pageant title, "Miss Hometown." Even though she now had very few teeth, we could see that she had been a beauty in her day. It was also evident that she was a tyrant in her day too. She would probably take no guff from anyone. She was pretty sharp, and through the years that I knew her, I saw very little deterioration in her condition. Marie could frequently be found in bed. Several times I was able to get her out of bed by bringing her Italian bread and butter, but she'd retreat to her bed right after. Marie couldn't relate to any of the residents on the floor, but she loved company. When she saw the group of us, she lit up and was happy to visit with us. She was very affectionate and always very grateful for any time we spent with her or anything we gave her. Marie was often very

186

lonely, too. She said she had two sons who never came to see her. She begged me to call one son on the phone and ask him to come. I did call but got no response. Marie had one very special interest: She enjoyed visiting with the men who came to the floor. When she saw a man in the hall, she'd follow him and would even pinch him where she shouldn't. Once, my friend Janet Fiene from Round Lake brought her co-worker Denise Rempert who had trained her dogs to visit nursing homes. I thought that perhaps Marie would be interested in the dogs, but she wasn't: She was more interested in chasing after Janet's son Parker who was only 14 years old at the time. She also loved a uniform. She was after one of the kinder-gartners' fathers who was a policeman.

Even though Marie wasn't interested in Denise's two large dogs, the other residents were very happy to see them when we took them to all the floors. The dogs were called Mickey (Disney's Mickey) and Charlie Brown – well-trained, very gentle, and happy to perform tricks with tennis balls. Mama was interested in the dogs for a brief moment but she had her Dukie. When Denise stopped to talk to Mama, Mama invited her over to the house for an Italian spaghetti dinner. Janet asked if she was invited too, but Mama told her to mind her own business and swore at her. We laughed because Mama had never seen Denise before, but Jan was around Mama a lot. While Jan and I were laughing, Marie, the beauty queen, was trying to talk dirty with Jan's son Parker. We intervened as quickly as we could. Always an interesting time at the home!

Laurie, the oldest person with Down Syndrome at the nursing home, was healthy, partially blind, and not verbal. She had a great sense of touch. She needed to be fed and her sense of taste always delighted her and she rewarded the aides with a big smile at mealtimes. She had a wonderful collection of stuffed animals that someone had given her. When Mickey and Charlie came visiting, she felt their soft fur and wet noses. It was the first time I saw her respond so warmly and with sounds of delight; she had made a connection. It made the dogs' visit to the home so worthwhile just to see the glow in Laurie.

Lorraine was always so neat, clean, and sweet, and she often sat quietly like such a lady. Although she was mobile, she was not usually noticed because of her quiet demeanor. But such a beautiful voice! Every time I saw her, I remembered that first day when I brought Mama to the home and she had sung the "Ave Maria." I always asked her to sing that hymn again for the friends I brought to visit and she moved us to tears every time. She prayed as she sang. Her husband visited her on the weekends and he rode a motorcycle. This led us to believe that in her day, Lorraine might have led a very adventurous life.

Carole wore several rosaries and necklaces around her neck and always had a purse in her hand. She was very warm and affectionate, always glad to see all those who greeted her, always inviting them to her mother's house. I first met Carole on a floor where the residents are very alert and oriented. In a short time she had deteriorated so quickly that she had to be placed on the Alzheimer's floor. With this disease, people often adopt a behavior reflective of something that was very important to them in their better days. Carole probably loved dressing up and going about town, because we would always find her racing down the hall, purse in hand and some fancy hat on her head.

Isabelle was quite sharp and although she was in a wheelchair, she would be allowed to go to another floor for Bingo. Mostly, she went there because she had a "crush" on the manager of the home. Isabelle filled me in on the new improvements to the building and anything she might have overheard when she was hanging out near the office. She had a brother and sister-in-law who came to visit her separately because they were divorced. Her brother gave her money for the Pepsi machine and for junk food treats. Isabelle was a large woman and I noticed that her clothes didn't fit her well, so TC and I collected our "old" clothes for her. These clothes made her feel very stylish and happy. For her birthday we sang songs in the hall and I brought her a big bottle of Pepsi as a treat. Isabelle was always sharp and had a great grasp of language. She always remembered me, and she liked Mama Rose. She got a kick out of the fact that Mama had Dukie. Sadly, she became very ill and had to be hospitalized. When she returned to the home, the Alzheimer's disease was more evident and she was more confused and no longer recognized me nor recalled the moments we had shared.

Gloria was as Irish as could be. TC could say something to her in Gaelic and that would bring a smile. She often giggled in delight when given compliments. I would sing "If You're Irish, Come into the Parlor" and she would join in the singing. Sometimes she would be having a bad day and would tell me to back off or scream at me, "You're no singer!" I'd laugh, continue to sing, and she'd join me anyway. Sometimes she fought with everyone in the dining room before meals, but even in those angry moods we couldn't help but like her. Gloria had a daughter who was a Sister of Providence and did Gloria's laundry several times a week. Gloria often said the Rosary with us and was really such a delightful person. She died at the age of 94, and I know she is happy with the Lord.

Rita was another sweetheart we came to love. She was in a wheelchair yet didn't have the sight to be very mobile. She had suffered through many illnesses that brought her close to death and was always so needy and would often cry for help. Rita would scream non-stop, "Help me, help me!" We figured out that she just wanted someone to hold her hand or talk with her. One day when a group of us were singing in the hall, Rita was screaming "Help me" and when I asked her what we could do for her, she said loudly, "I want to sing!" We wheeled her out to the hall to join us. It was a very rewarding moment. Rita had a twin who had died several years before and she longed to be united with her twin sister. We prayed with Rita and saw the comfort that this gave her. She finally did go peacefully to God.

Ellie was a feisty little lady about five feet tall whose feet didn't touch the floor in her wheelchair. She rolled around the floor telling everyone what to do and how to do it. She would chase me in her wheelchair and demand all my attention. When asked how she was, she always responded in such a way that we understood she seemed to be in a lot of physical pain, which is apparently what made her so cranky. However, within a few minutes I could get her laughing. She was 94 years old and quite sharp. She knew the words to all the songs and occasionally got a little tired of repeating the "Hail Mary" when she said the Rosary with us: "How many are we going to say?" she'd ask. She always questioned me as soon as I walked off the elevator, wanting to know where I had been and why I hadn't come sooner. When it was time for me to go home, I often had to sneak off to the elevator to leave or Ellie would claim my attention if she caught me, but on other days she'd just ask for a kiss and a hug and then give me permission to leave.

Judy was always pleasant and friendly, probably the most stable resident on the Alzheimer's floor. She said she had nine brothers, but I never saw her have a visitor. She would always be on a chair in the hall greeting folks. The only time I saw Judy get angry was on her birthday when I asked her age; she said she was 26 and waiting for her mom and dad. One of the staff told me Judy was 82 years old, but Judy said, "Where did you come up with a number like that?" Then Judy told me to mind my own business in a nasty manner. Judy was always with Irma. They were roommates and they looked out for each other. One night when Mama was not well, I stayed with her until after midnight. I saw Irma and Judy sitting in the hall, content just to be together. Finally, they came to Mama's room to ask if they could have a drink. I found some juice for them and they thought it was wine. "Why not have wine? We can get plowed," they said. "We're going to bed anyway!"

Most of the experiences I had were with the women because many of the men on the Alzheimer's floor were very quiet and stayed to themselves. Sadly, some were violent. But then there was our special friend Edgar, a little gentle man with a big smile that attracted everyone to him. He always wore a baseball hat or shirt. His son lived out of town, so Edgar's clothes were old and tattered. He had lost language skills so it was often hard to understand him. He loved to see the young children who visited and he was always looking for more cookies. The beauty queen told us she was very close friends with him and took showers with him but we knew this wasn't true. It made Edgar blush and all of us laugh when she talked like this. It was always delightful to see Edgar but then suddenly he became very ill. We all visited him and sat awhile with him. His son came in from out of town, but Edgar was in a semi-conscious state. It was evident that his son and daughter-in-law loved him very much and knew he had a cute personality. They hadn't seen him in a long time and didn't have the comfort of his smile or laughter now that he was so ill. Luckily, we had made a videotape of Mama with some of the folks we came to know and love. Edgar was one of them. We were so happy that we could share the tape with Edgar's son before his dad died. It brought tears of joy for him to see his father and to know we loved him too.

Sally was new to the home. On one of her first nights, obviously very afraid, she sat quietly in the recreation room in a fur jacket. Mary Kay and I made an effort to talk to her and then offered to put the T.V. on for her. She then turned to us and asked, "Could I have a beer too?"

Millie looked to be about 50 years old and had lived at the home for about 10 years. She had difficulty walking and so they would put her in a chair that she couldn't get out of easily. She would smile and sit quietly for hours. Because she had diabetes, I carefully kept track of any cookies I gave her on my visits. Millie didn't talk. Then one day I heard an aide say something to her and Millie repeated it. I tried the same thing and after that I could get her to repeat short phrases. She never initiated conversation, remaining in her silent world day in and day out, responding to visitors only with a smile. She did become excited if she were offered food. Once, my friend Sue visited the home and brought her cat "Ragmop," and Millie lit up with joy. After that, she would hold the cat and love it whenever Ragmop visited, and she wasn't about to share the cat with the other residents either. When Millie was sitting next to Mama Rose, she would sometimes take her food, so I started bringing Millie a milk shake of her own to eliminate this problem.

Gladys was quiet but very sharp, a resident looking out for the other residents. She chose to be on the Alzheimer's floor so she could be helpful. She was a diabetic and asked only that I pick up sugar-free candy for her from Dominick's so she could have it in her room when she wanted it. In return she would take good care of Mama. That was a fair deal and I was happy to buy her candy. She often joined us in praying the Rosary and conversing with the children who came to visit.

Margareta was a sweet Polish lady who smiled and spoke very little English. While she loved the children and would dance with them, she wasn't too nice to Mama. Margareta would push Mama out of her seat and try to take Dukie. I often had to intervene carefully.

Wilma was pretty sharp and walked the halls with Mama, although she wasn't fast enough to keep up with Mama Rose. I walked in one day to find Wilma non-verbal and staring into space. No one could say what happened. She no longer responded to my greetings or showed any recognition of her surroundings. She was no longer ambulatory either. The disease often works this quickly and it can be devastating.

There was Flo who often undressed in the hall. I often had to call a nurse to dress her. She talked a lot to the aides, especially to Ted, the male aide. She would throw things at Mama if she were sitting next to her and would try to get Mama's food. I often requested she not be seated next to Mama. When TC and I arrived one Sunday, the staff hadn't noticed that Flo had seated herself next to Mama, so I sat between them. She started throwing things at me, like napkins and silverware, and saying loudly, "You fat a-- from ------- all the men!" We laughed and TC added

"And I thought you were fat from eating too much!" It was a belly laugh moment for us. Flo's daughter was close by and so embarrassed that she left in tears. I tried to find her to tell her it was okay for I certainly understood the situation. But the incident did help me understand what a nurse had told me once, that most of the families didn't come because it was too embarrassing for them to see their family member act out.

Not all the residents were pleasant, of course. People with Alzheimer's can be difficult company. There were some ladies on the floor who would yell out obscenities and were not easy to be around. Annette would reach out to grab someone and wouldn't let go. She was moaning all the time. There was Charlene asking us to take her home to see her mom and dad. She kept looking for the bus, repeating this request non-stop all day. There was Helen, who was blind but not short on lung-power. She screamed non-stop for hours. Ellie would try to quiet her to no avail and the other ladies would tell her she was giving them a headache. There was Deanna who followed me around but never had anything to say. There was Anita who went into rages and refused to visit with her family. She screamed and fought with everyone. One day I came in to find that Anita had to be sedated to keep her calm after a terrible rage.

It was difficult to come for a visit and find that one of the residents had died the night before or had changed very rapidly. The staff was always very careful not to talk about the loss in front of the residents. We had the privilege of praying with some of the residents before they died. Mary Kay and I prayed with Jeannette before she died and Mary Kay also prayed with Robert before he passed away. We had a chance to say goodbye to our good friend Edgar before he died. I mourned the residents on

Mama's floor who passed away, for I had come to know almost all of them. I learned so much about life and death in that nursing home. I also was grateful that those who died were finally at peace now with the Lord.

Mary Kay Hastings
at Mama Rose's birthday celebration

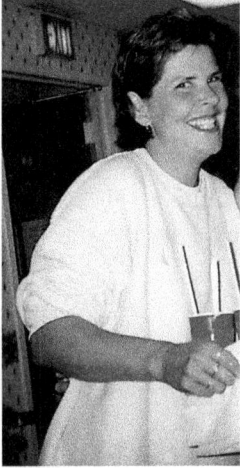

Mama Rose's birthday cake

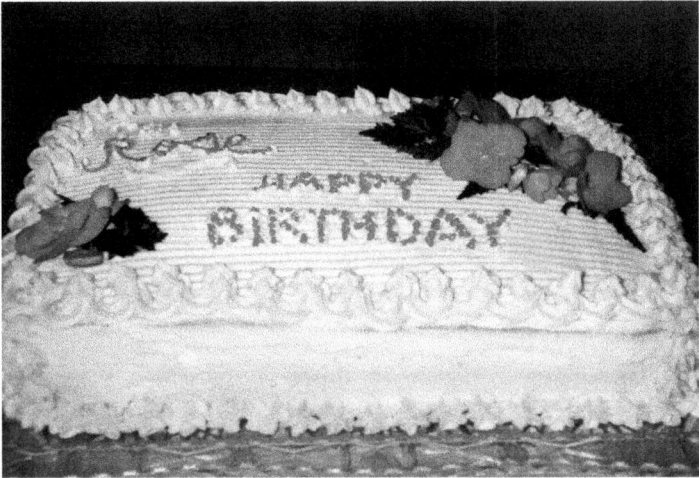

Mama Rose
at her nursing home birthday party

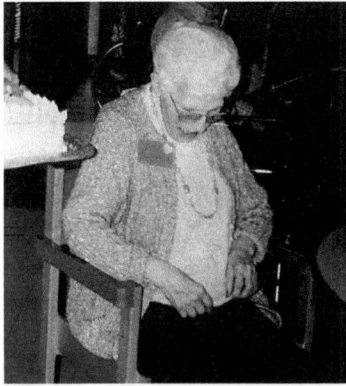

18

Mama's Final Days

I received a call at school one day that Mama had fallen down. Would I come to the home immediately after school? I was very concerned but in no way prepared for how I found her that afternoon. The staff had called the doctor to check her out and to give her something to calm her down. It had to be very frightening for her if she was aware of the fall. When I got there, she was in bed resting quietly. When I turned her over I was shocked to see that the whole side of her face was black and blue. It was a terrible sight. The doctor suspected that she had suffered a mini stroke and when she went down, she didn't know how to break her fall. I was concerned that these small strokes would increase her loss of brain tissue and speed up her lack of coordination. The staff were monitoring her walking, making sure she sat down to rest and giving her medication to ease any discomfort. Everyone was shocked to see her like this. When the manager saw her, and knowing Mama's sense of humor, he asked what the other guy looked like. The activity director felt so bad for Mama and went to see her as often as she could. It is very logical that the people will fall because of their lack of coordination caused by the deterioration from the disease, but I will never forget the sight of that bruise on her face. I had seen black and blue marks on other residents from falls, but none to this extent. Mama wasn't aware her face was bruised. It took several weeks for her face to look normal again. She did recover and was still going up and down the halls, but she was walking more slowly. It would be just terrible if Mama couldn't walk those halls. Sadly, this was the beginning of Mama's decline.

I didn't take Mama out of the home on little trips as often now since she was having such difficulty getting into the car and going up and down curbs and steps. But by Easter, Mama was all healed and ready for a celebration at my friend Mary Kay's home. Mary Kay bought a huge stuffed bunny for Mama to hold and talk to for the day. She was quieter than usual but very agreeable and pleasant for most of the visit. When it was time for Mama's birthday in June, I threw a big party at the home in the main dining room. I invited many of my Bunco friends as well as our usual visiting group. We had many hands to bring a number of the Alzheimer's floor residents down to the party. We had cake and ice cream, we sang songs, and as before, the highlight was singing "Happy Birthday" to Mama. She giggled with delight when we sang to her.

During that summer, I could take Mama down for the Mass that was offered at the home. We had to leave several times because she would start talking very loudly, disturbing those at the Mass. Every Sunday morning, Communion ministers from our local church, St. Stephen's, would come with Communion for Mama. My friend Kathy Bulger brought her Communion several times, too. On one visit, Mama took the host and said to

Kathy, "This is it? One little cookie?" Mama never meant to be disrespectful. In fact she used to go to daily Mass after she retired. But her question was just another indication that her perception of Holy Communion being the Body and Blood of Jesus was no longer clear. I know the Lord so understood this precious soul and saw the love Mama had cherished for Him all of her life.

There were more events to share that summer and more visits that were a lot of fun.

The next year was pretty much the same with many good times, and yet there was growing evidence of Mama's diminishing skills. She had two more mini strokes and another fall. The staff tried to keep her in a wheelchair to keep her from falling, but to no avail. She was a walker. I didn't want her tied to a chair, but it is true that as soon as they even tried to keep her stationary, she started to go downhill in spirit. It was time. I asked Father Carl Morello, longtime pastor of St. Paul of the Cross Parish, to come to give her the Last Rites. She had seen him very often at school and at Church. He asked Mama Rose if she knew who he was. She looked up at him and said," I don't know who the h--- you are."

On Palm Sunday, I was getting off the elevator and saw Mama trying to speak to one of the Communion ministers who brought Communion to the residents every week. I noticed she was having difficulty telling the minister that she wanted the Eucharist so I told him that yes she did. I spoke to the nurse afterward and it was evident that Mama had suffered another mini stroke, one that took away her speech. She still gave me a big smile, but there were no more words shared between us. After consulting with her doctor, I learned that she would also have difficulty swallowing food. This was the beginning of the end. Many times I told Mama it was all right for her to go to the Lord. I told her I was grateful for the time we had and all the love we shared. We hugged often and her smile was always there.

I received a call from the home the following night that she was very stressed and frightened. Mary Kay and I went to the home at midnight to calm her down. She was happy to see us and able to relax. After that I stayed with her each night because she seemed to fear the loneliness of the nighttime most of all. The nurses and the aides came in often at the end of their shift to say goodbye to Mama. Then when they returned a day or two later, they were surprised to see Mama still there and smiling. Our circle of friends came to visit and to laugh and talk around her bed so that she would be comforted. Mama didn't know what was going on but she seemed to enjoy having people around her. I'm sure the distractions made the time pass more quickly. Her stuffed Dukie was always at her side. Throughout this whole week, Holy Week, Mama was only able to get some water down. The supervisor couldn't believe how strong Mama was during this time even though she was losing weight and very frail.

***

Mama Rose went to be with the Lord on April 12, 1998. She died on Easter Sunday with a smile on her face and Dukie at her side.

"You Are My Sunshine" sings forever in my heart.

Mama Rose on Palm Sunday.
She went to be with the Lord
on Easter Sunday, April 12, 1998.

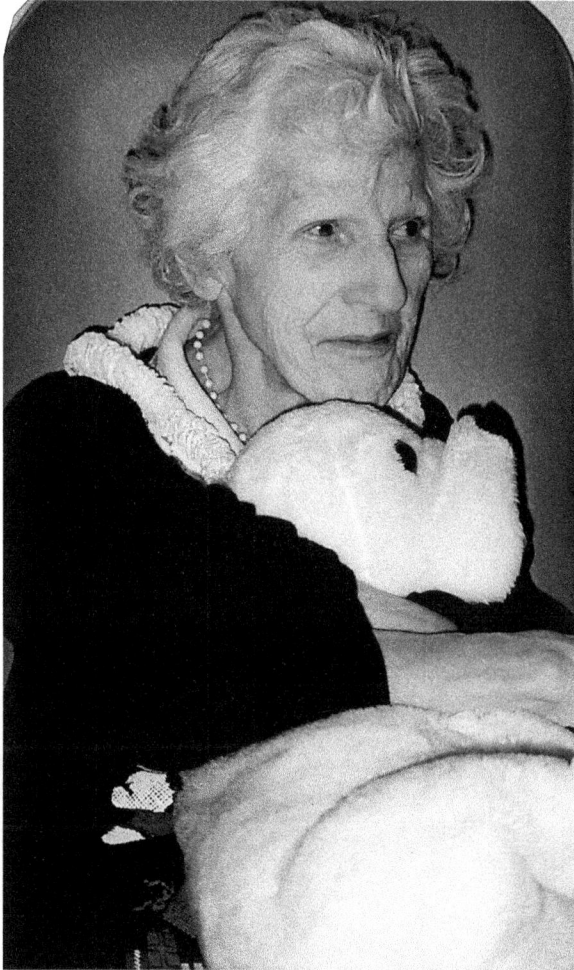

Acknowledgments

It is a pleasure to thank the many people whose encouragement and support make this writing possible.

First, I am grateful to God who gave me a wonderful Mama to love all of my life. I'm grateful that I could be the caregiver for my mother as she agonized through the devastating disease of Alzheimer's.

My husband Richard was so supportive of my caregiving. This enabled me to extend loving care for Mama during the last years of her life.

The caregiver needs much support and that support came from my many friends. My dear friend Mary Therese Pallasch (TC) was there daily with whatever was needed—sometimes just a phone call.

Another wonderful friend was Jane Schaible who gave me helpful advice through her insights and experience with the demands of caregiving and the search for services.

I am grateful to so many families who were generous in numerous ways, and I will always remember my dear friends who helped me care for Mama when she was still living in my home: Laurene Moran, Lynn Gentile, Betty Weiss, Terri Servedio, and my friends from my Bunco group. I know I'm forgetting many folks who were there to help, to support.

The St. Paul of the Cross Parish family—the Hastings, the Whalens, Donna Cornille, Sister Lois M. Rossi of the Franciscan Sisters of Chicago, Sister Anne Michelle LaMarre of the Sisters of Loretto, Pat Meyer, Nancy Okerstrom, Barbara Stavnem, Sue Battaglia, Kathy Bulger, Maria Pohlson, Sue Kilmer, and so many wonderful friends—they were all there with strong support. And thanks to all the Heckmans who helped me see this book in print.

I also thank the parents who were so generous in allowing me to bring their children to the nursing home. Groups of kindergartners and eighth graders brought so much joy to the folks who lived there.

Others were so generous in helping me, such as John Zielinski and his daughter Jenny, and Sister Kathleen, a Franciscan Sister of Chicago.

If I missed your name, know that I am forever grateful for all you did for Mama and for the love you gave her. Last, but not least, thanks to the staff of the nursing home who took such good care of Mama during the last two years of her life.

Family Photos

Mama Rose at Uncle Carmen's wedding.

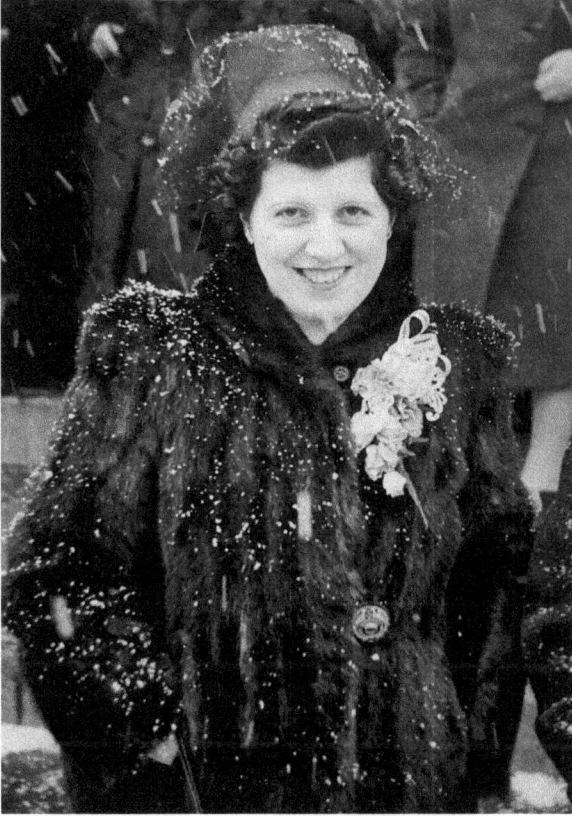

Mama Rose with Camille at the park.

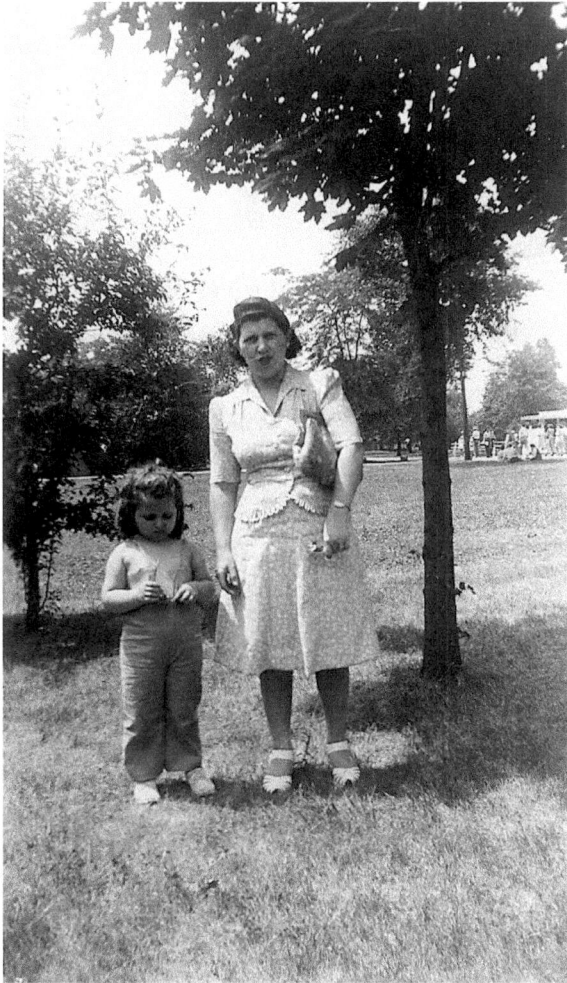

Camille and Mama Rose shopping downtown.

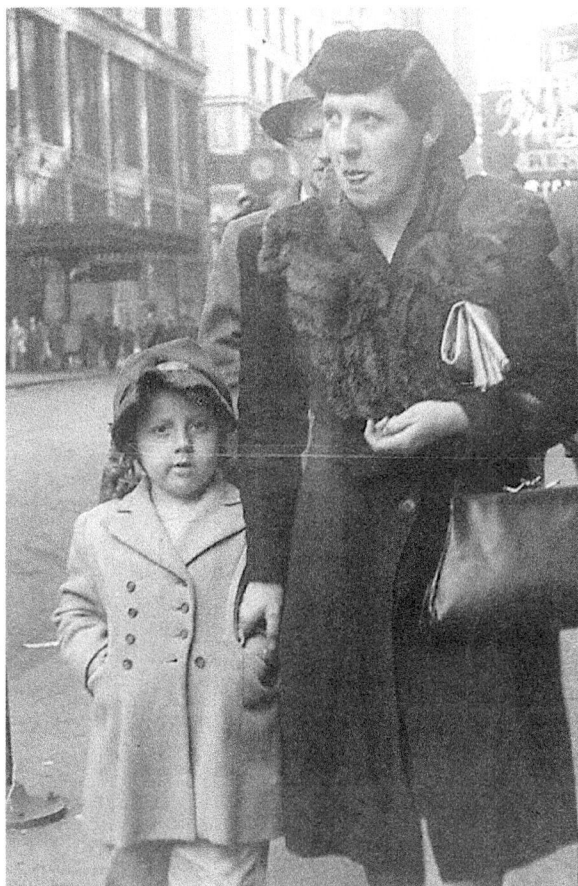

Camille enters the Sisters of Mercy as a postulant.

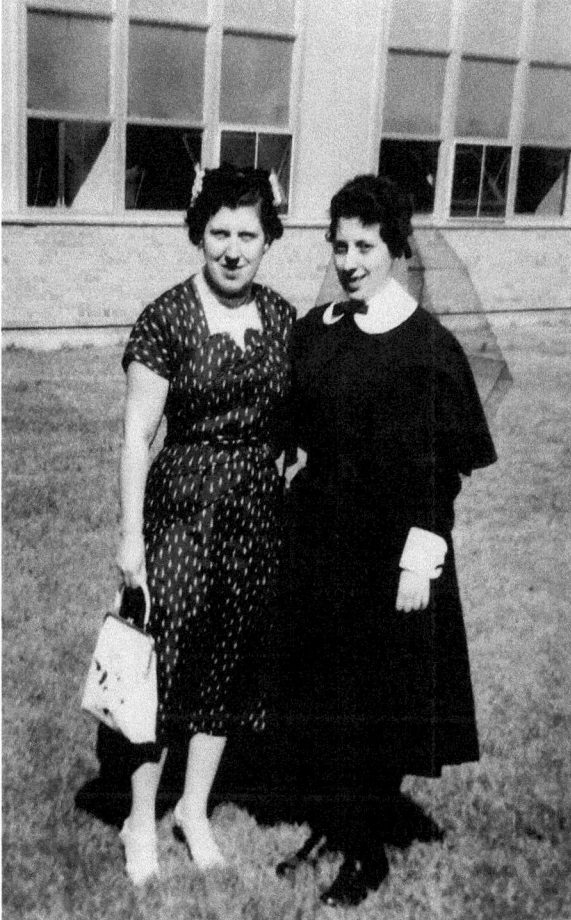

*Mama Rose visits the convent
when Camille is a novice.*

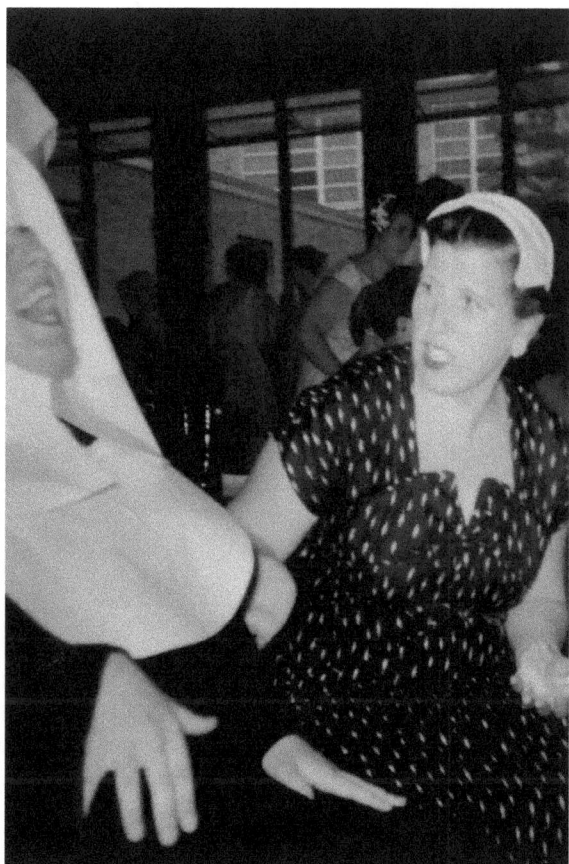

Mama Rose and Camille on the day of Camille's profession of vows. She wears a new simplified habit.

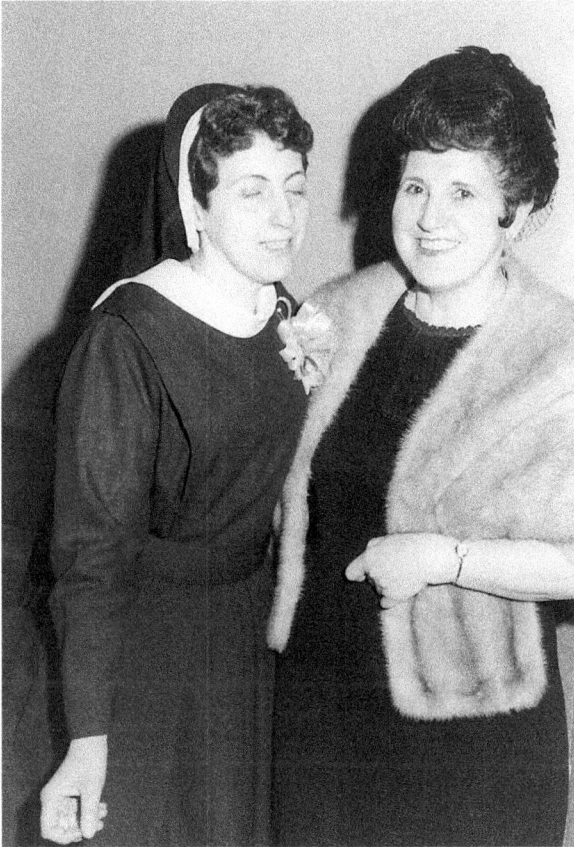

At Como Inn party after Camille's profession of vows.

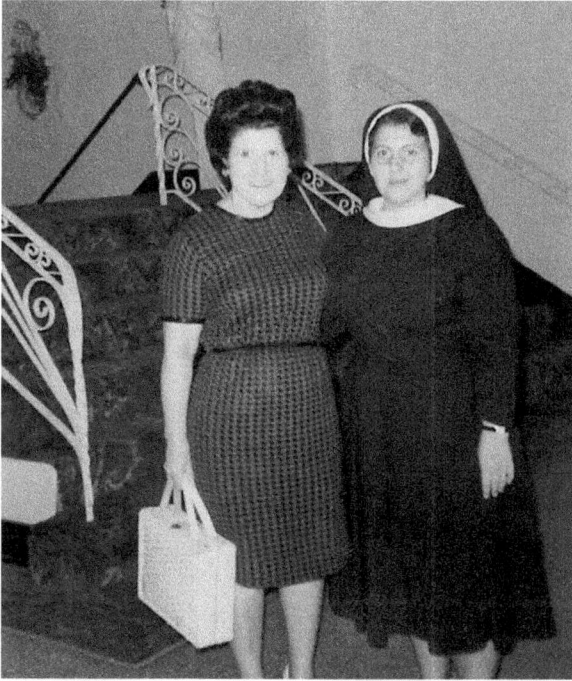

Mama Rose in Hawai'i.

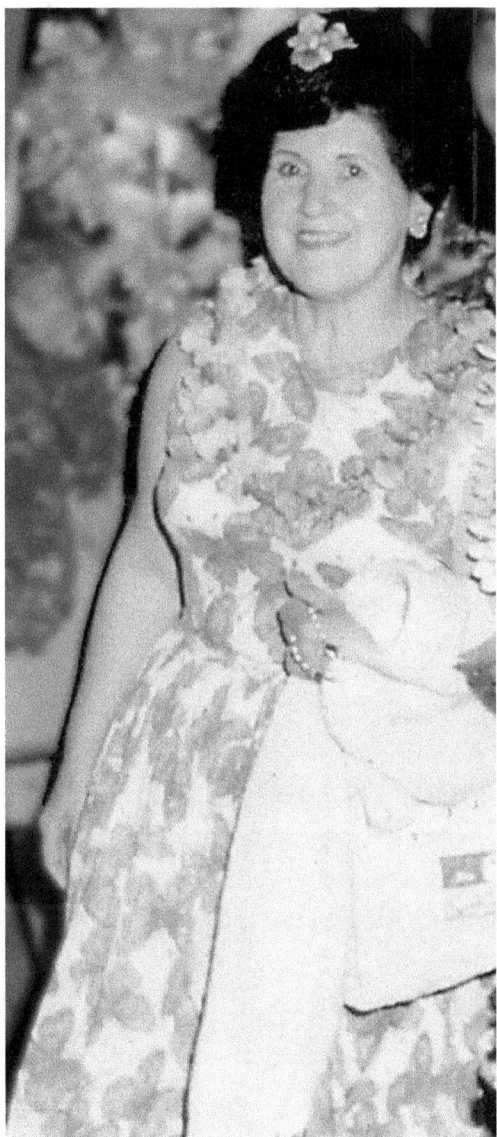

Nicki and Mama Rose.

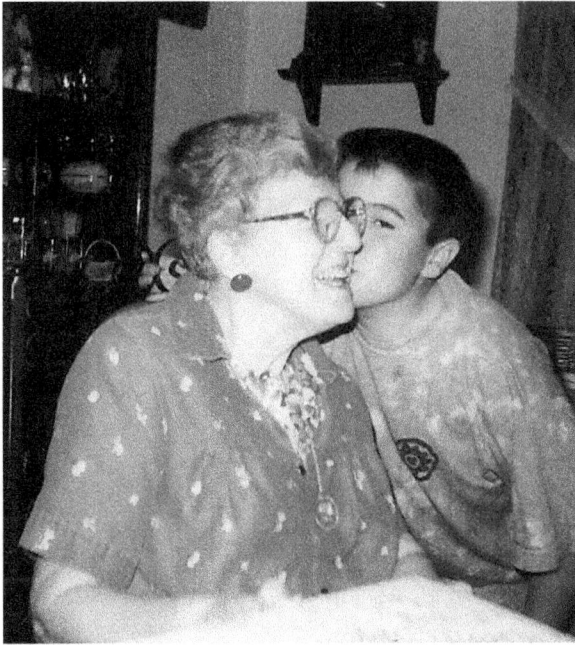

Mama Rose, Mary Therese Pallasch (TC),
and Camille at Pheasant Run for the weekend

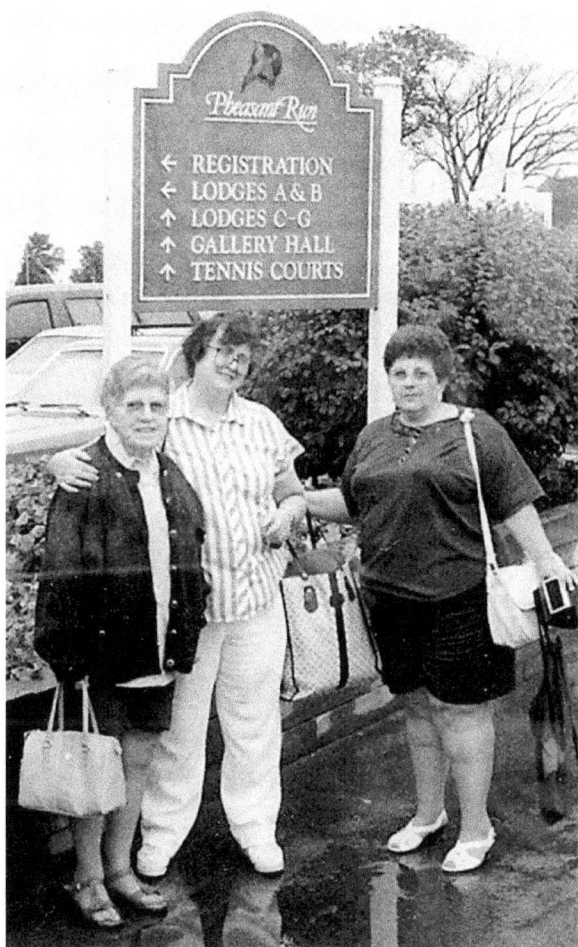

Mama Rose and Nancy Okerstrom playing Bunco.

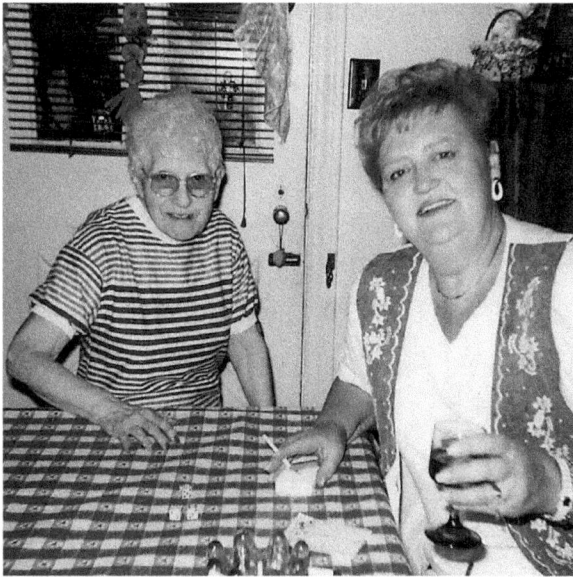

Pat Meyer and Nancy Okerstrom at Bunco.

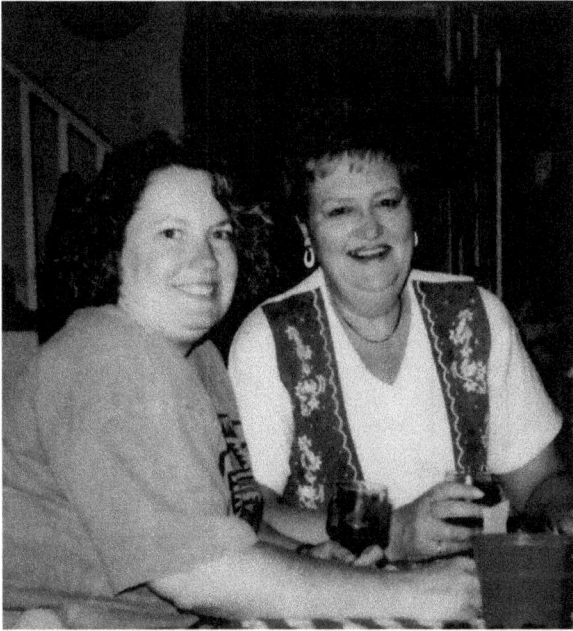

Mama Rose and Richard with Hershey.

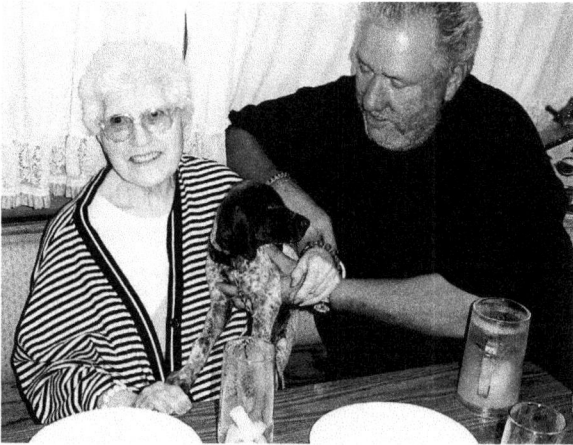

Mama Rose and Brooklyn (Duke II).

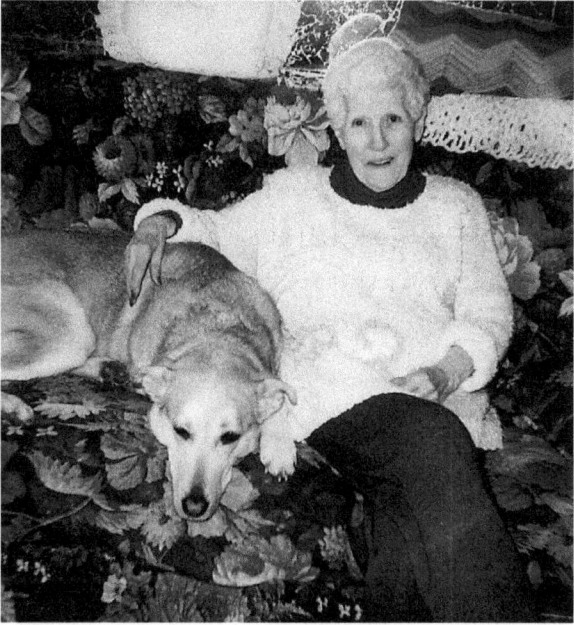

Mama Rose with the Gentiles' dog.

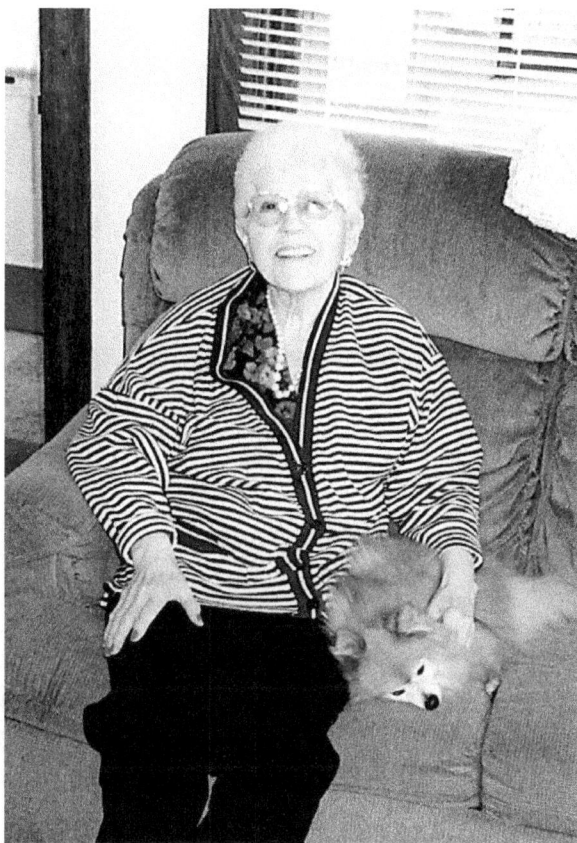

*Mama Rose and Camille
at the St. Joseph Table,
St. Paul of the Cross*

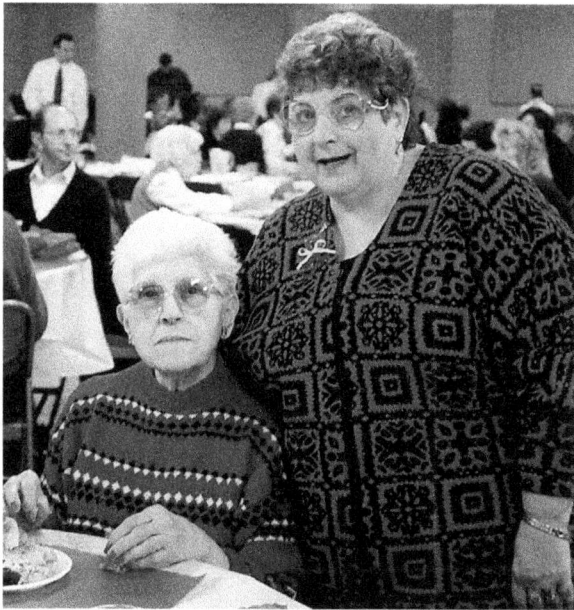

Our Santa.

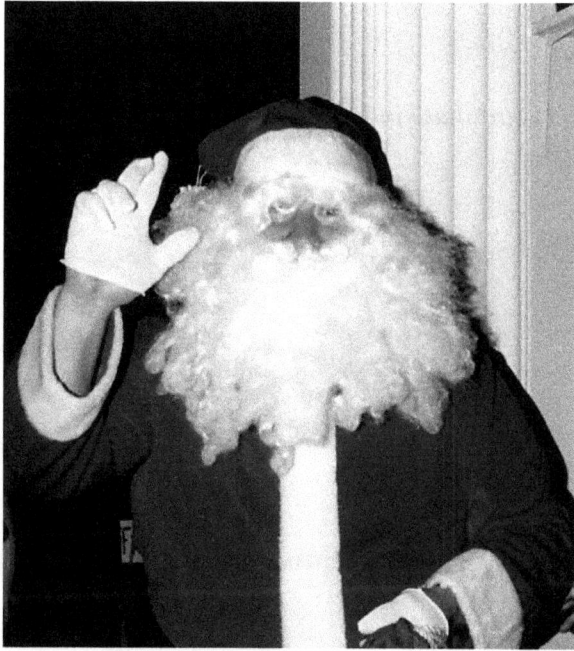

Santa at kindergarten party with Jane.

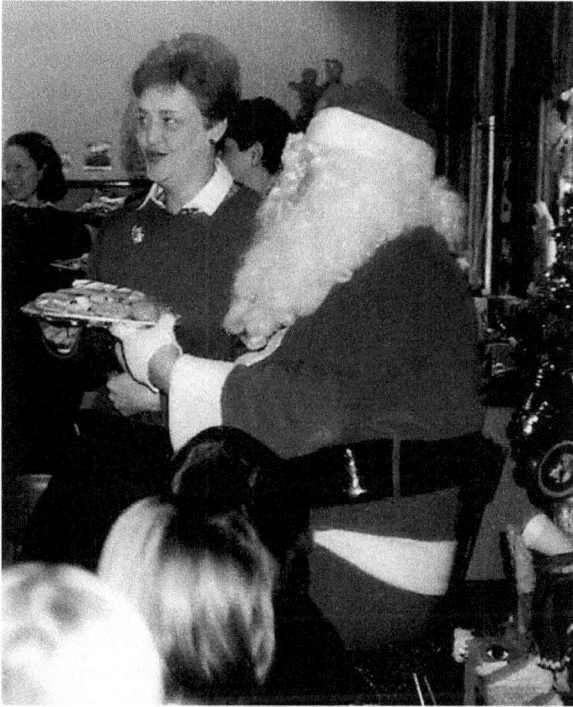

Mama Rose with her milkshake.

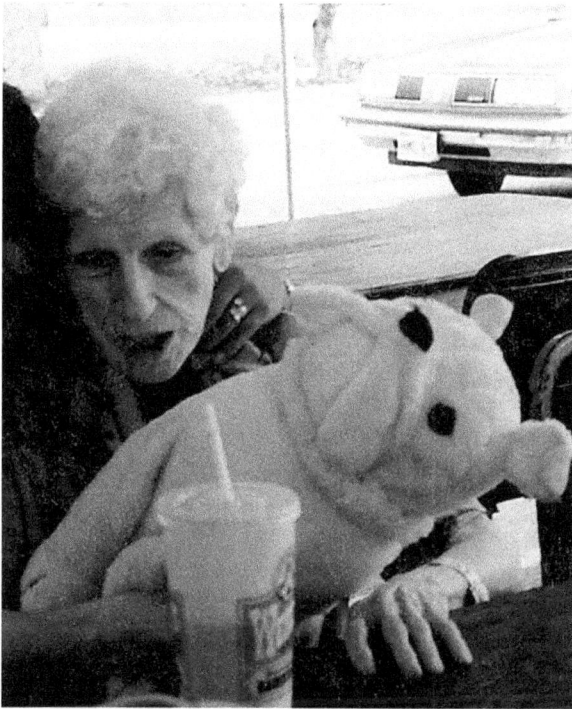

Camille, Mama Rose, and Dukie.

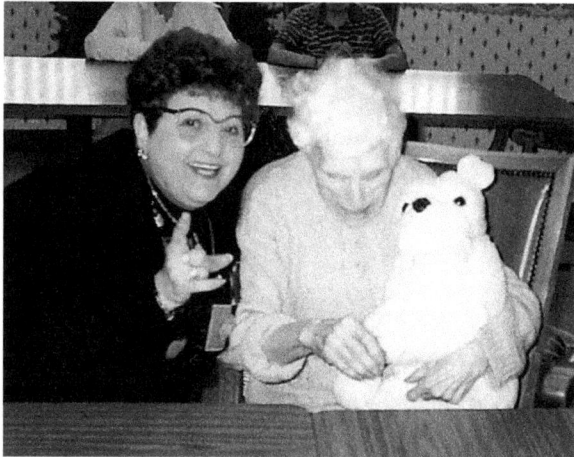

*The Easter Bunny (Mary Kay Hastings)
and Camille visit the nursing home.*

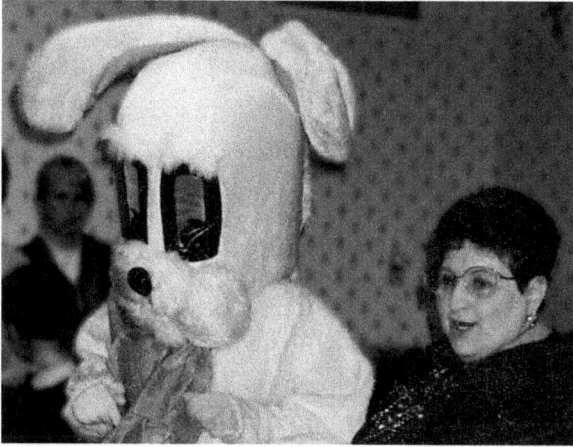

About the Author

A lifelong resident of the Chicago area, Camille Grafer is a retired elementary school teacher who wrote this memoir to honor her mother Rose. Camille lives in the northwest suburbs with her husband Richard.

www.ingramcontent.com/pod-product-compliance
Lightning Source LLC
Chambersburg PA
CBHW062347300326
41947CB00013B/1511